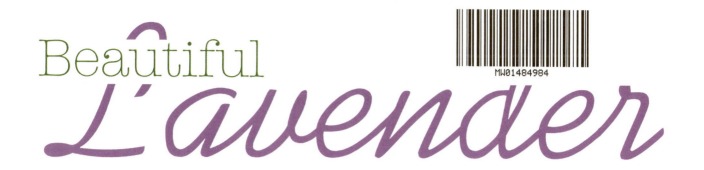

Beautiful L'avender

A GUIDE AND WORKBOOK FOR GROWING, USING, AND ENJOYING LAVENDER

By Janice Cox

MW01484984

Enjoy!
Janice Cox

1503 S.W. 42nd St.
Topeka, KS 66609-1265, USA
Telephone: (785) 274-4300
Fax: (785) 274-4305
www.ogdenpubs.com

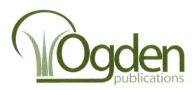

First Edition. Copyright © 2020 Ogden Publications
All rights reserved

Text © 2020 Janice Cox
Photography © 2020 Janice Cox
Additional Photography, see Page 112

No part of this book may be reproduced in any form without written permission of the copyright owners. All images in this book have been reproduced with the knowledge and prior consent of the artist concerned, and no responsibility is accepted by producer, publisher, or printer for any infringement of copyright, or otherwise, arising from the content of this publication. Every effort has been made to ensure that credits accurately comply with the information supplied. We apologize for any inaccuracies that may have occurred and will resolve inaccurate or missing information in a subsequent reprinting of the book.

Publisher: Bill Uhler
Editorial Director: Christian Williams
Merchandise and Event Director: Andrew Perkins
Production Director: Bob Cucciniello
Special Content Group Editor: Jean Teller
Special Content Assistant Editors: Blair Gordon, Eli Hoelscher, Kalli Jo Smith
Book Design and Layout: Amanda Barnwell

Ogden Publications titles are also available for retail, wholesale, promotional, and bulk purchase. For details, contact Customer Service: (800) 234-3368; customerservice@ogdenpubs.com; or Ogden Publications, Inc., 1503 S.W. 42nd St., Topeka, Kansas 66609-1265.

ISBN: 978-1-948734-18-9

Printed in the U.S.A.

Acknowledgements

To my grandmother, Ruth Campbell, who first introduced me to beautiful lavender. I think of you often. And to my granddaughter, Campbell Marie McDermott, I intend to teach you all about lavender, and you can use up all my bath products!

Thank you to my husband, Ray, and daughters Lauren and Marie, who are always there to hear my ideas, try a new recipe, and help with photos.

Thank you to my agent, Laurie Harper, for her support and friendship. Thank you to Christian Williams, Andrew Perkins, and Randy Smith at Ogden Publications for helping me with the business side of creating and selling a book.

Many thanks to the best creative team at Ogden Publications. You are all amazing and my favorites! Jean Teller, Amanda Barnwell, Blair Gordon, Eli Hoelscher, and Kalli Smith. I have loved working with all of you.

We are all born with a natural beauty, it is how we use it that makes us beautiful. You are all beautiful!

Janice Cox is the author of *Beautiful Luffa, Natural Beauty for All Seasons, Natural Beauty at Home,* and *Natural Beauty from the Garden.*

This book belongs to the garden library of:

_____

Table of Contents

NOTE: The recipes and treatments contained in this book are generally safe and effective. However, despite every effort to offer expert advice, it is not possible for this book to predict an individual person's reaction to a particular recipe or treatment. The reader should consult a qualified physician. Neither the publisher, Ogden Publications, nor the author, Janice Cox, accepts responsibility for any effects that may arise from following the recipes or treatments and using the products from the recipes in this book.

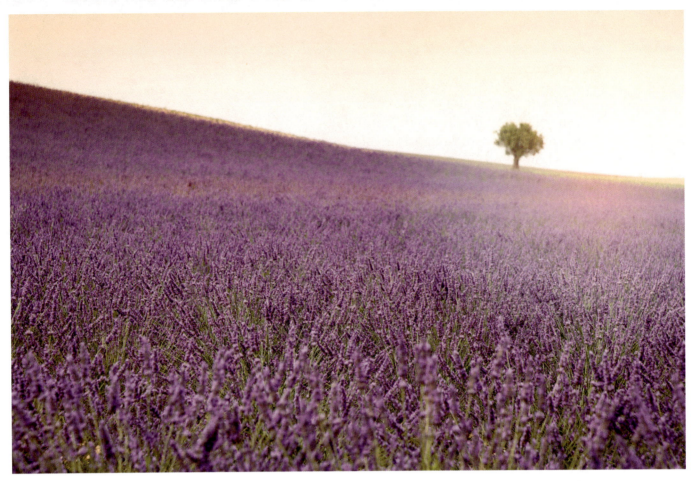

Introduction

I love lavender! In fact, it was probably the first herb that I remember using, long before I even knew what an herb was. My grandmother first introduced me to the scent at a very young age. I loved to take long bubble baths at her house because she had these Yardley English Lavender bath tablets that came in an elaborate gift box with a purple grosgrain ribbon. The ribbon opened a small cardboard drawer where fragrant bath tablets were individually wrapped in gold foil. She had drawers and cupboards full of products and samples, but it is those lavender tables that I remember best. When I unwrapped their gold foil and dropped them in the tub, they fizzed and danced in the warm bathwater. To me, this was beauty magic, and I loved it!

It wasn't until I was much older, and experimenting with my own collection of cosmetic products and recipes, that I truly understood the point of these products, or even how the scent of lavender could be used to calm the body and the mind. My recipe for Lavender Bath Bombs on Page 56 is my attempt to recreate those lavender tablets and their bath magic.

When I put together my first book, *Natural Beauty at Home*, lavender was a key ingredient in many of my body-care recipes and treatments, because it is one of the most fragrant and versatile herbs, especially when it comes to body care. The word lavender even comes from the Latin verb *lavare*, which means to wash. If you shop the aisles of your local drugstores or natural food stores, you will see a number of products featuring this fragrant herb. It is one of the most popular key cosmetic ingredients for its relaxing scent, and also for its anti-bacterial and anti-inflammatory properties. You will find lavender featured in nearly every body-care product, as well as in skin- and hair-care lines.

As a culinary ingredient, lavender adds sophistication that elevates the most basic of recipes. Whether added to sweet or savory dishes, lavender is just as versatile as other popular herbs such as mint, marjoram,

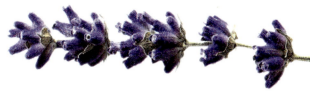

thyme, and rosemary. Classic lavender recipes include shortbread cookies, scones, and herbes de Provence seasoning mixes. The flavor of lavender can be used to enhance other common products such as cheeses, beer, cake mixes, and cocktails. It has been enjoyed as a fragrant tea for centuries. Queen Victoria was well-known for regularly enjoying a cup of lavender tea and using it as a cosmetic product. In fact, she used Yardley London products just like my grandmother.

Lavender is also useful in the home. It repels bugs and insects, and it can be made into an effective linen spray or used in closet sachets and hangers to protect natural fabrics. Its anti-bacterial properties help you avoid harmful and toxic ingredients while cleaning your home naturally. You can even create a powerful cleaner for your chicken coop using Lavender Vinegar (see Page 43).

In fact, this ancient herb is now more popular than ever before. To demonstrate this, I decided to shop for as many lavender products as I could find at my local grocery store. After going up and down all the aisles, I had a full cart of products. Of course, I had a collection of bath salts, lotions, soaps, teas, and cookies. I also found lavender in products I had never even thought of: soda, beer, cheese, baby wipes, laundry detergent, and even cat litter. Lavender was featured in just about every aisle, and I live in a small town! That is probably why lately everything seems to smell like lavender. Also as I travel around the country speaking, I see more and more lavender being used. Several of my hotels have had a small vial of lavender spray next to the bed, designed to help guests wind down naturally and sleep well. I even stayed at one hotel in Arizona where they had bowls of dried lavender buds and small fabric bags in the lobby for making your own dream pillows. This workbook too has resulted from lavender's popularity; it grew out of a talk I have given all around the United States. It

has been so popular that, for one event in particular, MOTHER EARTH NEWS Fairs, they even added hands-on workshops and events at local lavender farms.

I hope this workbook provides you with the opportunity to discover more about growing and incorporating lavender into your everyday life. Of course, you don't have to grow your own lavender. It is easily found at most natural food stores and markets. Many lavender farms offer products and have U-pick events where you can bring home fresh lavender you've harvested yourself.

Your garden is the ultimate health spa. It has been scientifically proven that people who regularly go outdoors and work with plants are happier, healthier, and less stressed. Plants make us beautiful. Enjoy your plants, enjoy your garden, and enjoy yourself. You are beautiful!

Lavender

The *Lavandula* genus comprises almost 40 species of lavender; of those species, more than 400 varieties exist. Lavender is a member of the square-stem herb family, along with mint, sage, horehound, thyme, and marjoram. If you look closely at a sprig of lavender, you will see that the stems have four sides and look almost square in shape.

Lavender is a Mediterranean plant and loves full sun, and well-drained, almost-dry soil. The plant is native to Provence, France, famous for its lavender fields. However, because of its popularity, you can now find lavender growing all over the world. As a perennial, lavender will live more than two years, with an average life span of 3 to 5 years. However, I have heard of plants, if well cared for and under the right growing conditions, that have lasted up to 10 or 12 years. Lavender is a hardy plant and really does not suffer from many bothersome pests. It thrives in dry, hot conditions, so when you hear of people losing their plants, it is usually

Yardley London

Yardley London, or simply "Yardley's," as it is often called, is one of the most well-known lavender cosmetic companies. Found in 1770 by the Cleaver family, it is one of the oldest cosmetic companies. The company was purchased by William Yardley in 1823 and renamed Yardley London. Their signature scent, English Lavender (*Lavandula angustifolia*), grows in southern England. The company still exists today and is owned by a wealthy British family from India. They have branched out with other scents and products, but their lavender soaps and body-care products still remain their most popular. I often see them sold here in the United States in drugstores and even some grocery stores, and can't help but buy a bar of soap or two. The scent brings me back to my childhood.

because the plants have gotten too wet. Such conditions can cause rot or fungus, which are the usual reasons most plants die.

As a landscape plant, lavender can be planted as a border or grouped with other plants. Because they are drought-tolerant, they're ideal for planting in areas that do not get a lot of water. I have seen deer nibble on lavender, though they often leave it alone. Lavender is also fire-resistant. So if you live in the country or where forest fires are a threat, you may want to consider adding lavender in your landscape plan.

I'm often asked which lavender variety to choose, or what lavender will grow best in someone's yard. My best advice is to talk to experts in your area, such as local farmers and gardeners who are actually growing different varieties. Not every type of lavender will grow in every hardiness zone. In fact, I have even heard of varieties that thrive where they shouldn't.

I have found the best way to choose lavender plants and successfully grow them is to talk with your local nurseries and extension services. Joining organizations or visiting websites also help you garner valuable information for your county or state. I am a member of the United States Lavender Growers Association (USLGA) and The Oregon Lavender Association (OLA). You do not need to be a lavender farmer or professional to join these groups, and they provide a wealth of information from experienced members (see more info on Page 11).

Another way to see and learn about different varieties for your area is to attend a lavender festival. These festivals usually take place during the summer months when lavender is in full bloom. Farms and groups will host festivals that feature food, crafts, educational talks, music, and lots of fresh lavender. Many farms feature U-pick activities where, for a small fee, you can fill a bag or basket with fresh lavender to take home and enjoy.

The three main groups of lavender are English lavender (*Lavandula angustifolia*), French lavender (*L. dentata*), and Spanish lavender (*L. stoechas*). English lavender is probably the most popular and versatile, as it can be used for landscaping, in the bath, in the home, and as a culinary herb. It has several varieties, some even with pink or white flowers.

French lavender can be identified by its usually jagged leaves. These lavenders are well-known for their oil content and are popular for creating scented oils and hydrosols. Spanish lavender looks like it has wings or ears on the top of the flower bud. These plants too have a high oil content and were some of the first lavenders used by the Romans. However, their scent does not smell as sweet as the English and French varieties. This variety smells more like camphor, so they are usually used as landscape plants to attract pollinators. Some varieties of lavender have scented leaves with no flower buds at all.

With so many different varieties of lavender, you are sure to find one that suits your yard. They also can be grown in containers, and grow nicely in spots that get full sun.

Popular Lavender Varieties

Each variety of lavender has its own unique flowers, scent, and size. In some states, you may be able to grow several varieties, especially if you have mild winters and hot summers. In colder climates, your choices may be limited to hardier varieties. Experiment with plants that work best for you. The best way is to observe local plants and talk with other growers in your area.

Look to see if you have "microclimates" in your own garden. These are areas that may be warmer because of large rocks or concrete, which are warmed by the sun, absorbing heat to increase the area's temperature. I know the area along the backside of my house, which is in direct sunlight and near a concrete patio, always seems a bit warmer than the rest of my yard. I have a few lavender plants in pots there, and they do really well.

When choosing a variety, consider how you are going to use the plants. Are they for landscaping and to attract pollinators to your yard? Do you want to cook with the dried buds or create your own body-care products? Do you just love lavender and want to use the fresh flowers in your home? Knowing how you want to use them will help in deciding which variety to plant. Here are a few popular, successful varieties for most growers.

LAVANDULA ANGUSTIFOLIA: Usually called English lavender, this species is probably the most popular of all the varieties, as it grows well in most gardens and can survive cold winters. It also dries easily and has a lovely scent that can be

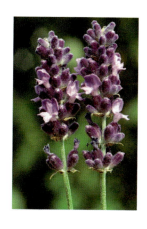

used as both a culinary herb and cosmetic herb. There are several different cultivars that vary in color and size. Some even have white and pink blooms, which are a nice surprise from the traditional purple.

LAVANDULA INTERMEDIA: 'Provence' and 'Grosso' are two of the most popular varieties of lavandins because of their long stems and oil-rich flower heads. Their scent may be a bit more camphor-like, but their buds are easy to dry and will keep their scent for a long time. This group of lavandins (hybrid lavenders cultivated for essential oil) is a good 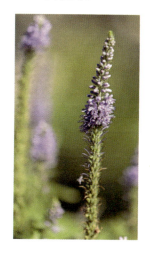 choice. If you are interested in making your own essential oils, 'Grosso' is easy to work with. It is also popular for making Lavender Wands (see Page 89) because of the variety's long, pliable stems.

LAVANDULA STOECHAS: Often called Spanish lavender, these plants look like little butterflies attached to the flower heads, and are usually used as landscape pollinator plants to attract the butterflies 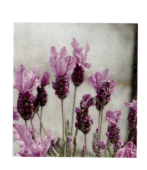 they resemble, as well as bees and other pollinators. These subtly scented lavender varieties are some of the first to bloom in the spring, though they are neither used for culinary nor cosmetic purposes.

9

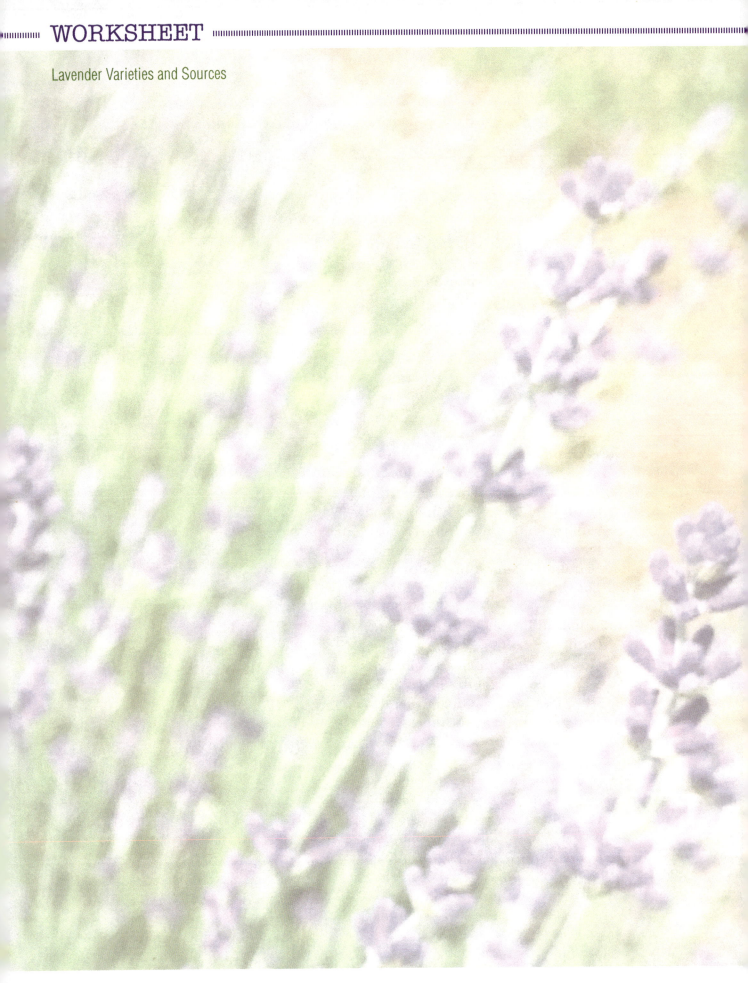

WORKSHEET

Lavender Varieties and Sources

The History of Lavender

Lavender is one of the oldest and most beloved herbs throughout history. I feel we all have a lavender story or memory. For me, it was my grandmother's soap. For others, it may be a garden spot or the scent of freshly washed linens. Lavender and its use dates back to ancient Egypt and is even mentioned in the Bible. It has been used throughout history for everything from mummification to the backdrop for a modern-day French fashion runway show. Lavender farms are popping up all over the world and have become popular stops for travelers looking for both culinary and wellness products and activities.

Lavender was first used in ancient times by Roman soldiers as a way to scent their bathwater and also keep their bodies healthy. Throughout history, healers and doctors have utilized the natural health benefits of plants; lavender is always mentioned because of its ability to heal the body while calming the mind. The Greeks used lavender to treat headaches and also heal minor cuts and burns.

Women who did the laundry in medieval England were often called "lavenders," because they used lavender-scented water when washing clothes and linens. The German nun and herbalist Hildegard von Bingen was well-known for her use of lavender water mixed with alcohol to treat headaches. Hildegard may have been one of the first herbal mixologists for her use of herbs, gin, vodka, and brandy. If you care to enjoy a lavender cocktail, see my recipes on Page 78. More on Hildegard can be found on the next page.

There is also a bit of magic or superstition around lavender in certain cultures. In Europe, lavender is often thrown on floors or into burning fires to

USLGA

The United States Lavender Growers Association (USLGA) was formed to support and promote the lavender industry, providing wealth of information on all things lavender. There are several levels of membership, and you do not need to be a lavender farmer or grower to become a member. I am what they call a "friend of lavender." The USLGA maintains a website and hosts a conference every two years that is both educational and inspirational. I attended my first one in Charleston, South Carolina, and was impressed with the speakers and activities. Most importantly, joining helps you network with growers in your area. Most states also have their own organizations that share the same mission of the USLGA to promote the enjoyment of lavender. I am a member of the Oregon Lavender Association, which has helped me with my own plants and also taught me several new ways to use them.

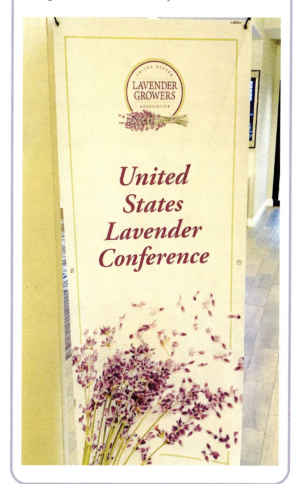

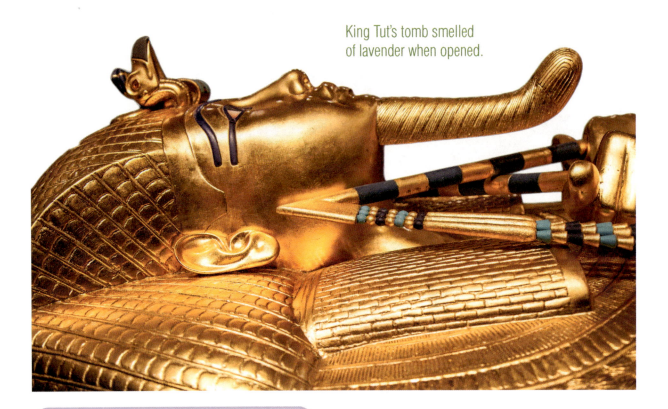

King Tut's tomb smelled of lavender when opened.

Hildegard von Bingen

I first discovered Hildegard von Bingen while researching an article on hops, which was the herb of the year for 2018. This amazing woman was born into a noble family in Germany, who gave her to the church when she was 8 years old. She never stopped learning, and became a physician, writer, and composer. She also loved plants, especially lavender, which she wrote about quite often. She advised readers to stay healthy by drinking warm wine infused with lavender. She passed away at the age of 76, and remains most well-known for her book, *The Book of Divine Love.*

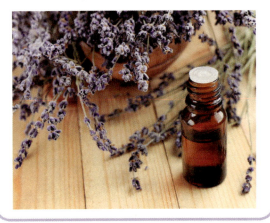

ward off evil spirits. In Italy, it was once customary to pin a sprig of lavender onto children's shirts as protection. In 1922, when Howard Carter opened up King Tutankhamun's tomb, the first aroma he smelled was lavender. Discovering the use of lavender in a pharaoh's tomb exemplifies how important this herb was in ancient Egypt.

Another royal, Queen Elizabeth I of England, loved lavender. She drank lavender tea and ate jam and cookies all made from the fragrant flower buds. Such treats can be found at most tea shops around the world.

The scent of lavender is one of the oldest perfumes in England, and during the Victorian era it was known as a "cure-all" plant. During World War II, a water-based cleaner containing lavender essential oil was used to disinfect and clean hospitals, while keeping patients calm and comfortable.

Distilled fresh lavender and lavender essential oil have long been used in aromatherapy practices. Lavender oil can be used to treat headaches, depression,

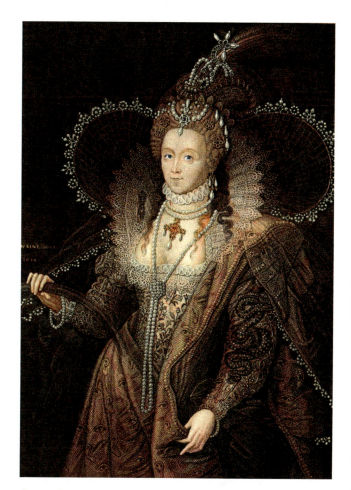

Queen Elizabeth I enjoyed lavender in her tea and cookies.

and anxiety. Lavender essential oil is still useful today; I have even seen little vials sold in airports to help people ease their fear of flying, or relax after a long day of travel. In France, people make hatbands from fresh lavender to wear while working in the garden. This helps ward off insects and also is believed to prevent headaches caused by the hot sun.

Today, with more and more people being interested in natural health and wellness, I am not surprised by the popularity of this useful plant. It is a plant we can all relate to because it represents nostalgia, health, and relaxation. It is also a plant that is easy to grow and can be used in a variety of ways. I have read that there are more than 100 uses for lavender, and I believe it. I have tried to include many of the more popular uses in this workbook. Feel free to create your own list on any of the blank pages at the end of each chapter.

Aromatherapy

Aromatherapy is a holistic practice that uses aromatic essential oils from plants to treat the body, mind, and spirit. Believed to enhance both physical and emotional health, this practice has been used by several ancient cultures around the world. The term "aromatherapy" was created by French perfumer and chemist René-Maurice Gattefossé in a book he wrote and published in 1937. He also wrote about the healing potential of lavender, especially for treating intense burns. Today, aromatherapy has become a household term, and products that work via the sense of smell will often use the term as part of their label. Essential oils and plant essences are featured in body-care products, home diffusers, and sprays. These oils have several benefits and make different health claims, from improving sleep quality to killing bacteria. Lavender is a popular and easy-to-find essential oil. It is sold almost everywhere, usually at natural food stores and drug stores in the skin-care section. Those who practice aromatherapy will say that every home should have a bottle of lavender essential oil. It has multiple uses as a natural anti-bacterial, antiseptic, antidepressant, sedative, and detoxifier. I will say as a note of caution: If you are sensitive or have not used essential oils, consult with your health practitioner or physician before using. I also want to point out that you should never ingest essential oils. I know there are some people who may disagree with me, but these are concentrated plant oils intended to be diluted in a carrier such as water, alcohol, or oil, and are intended for external use only.

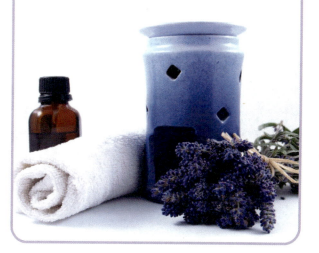

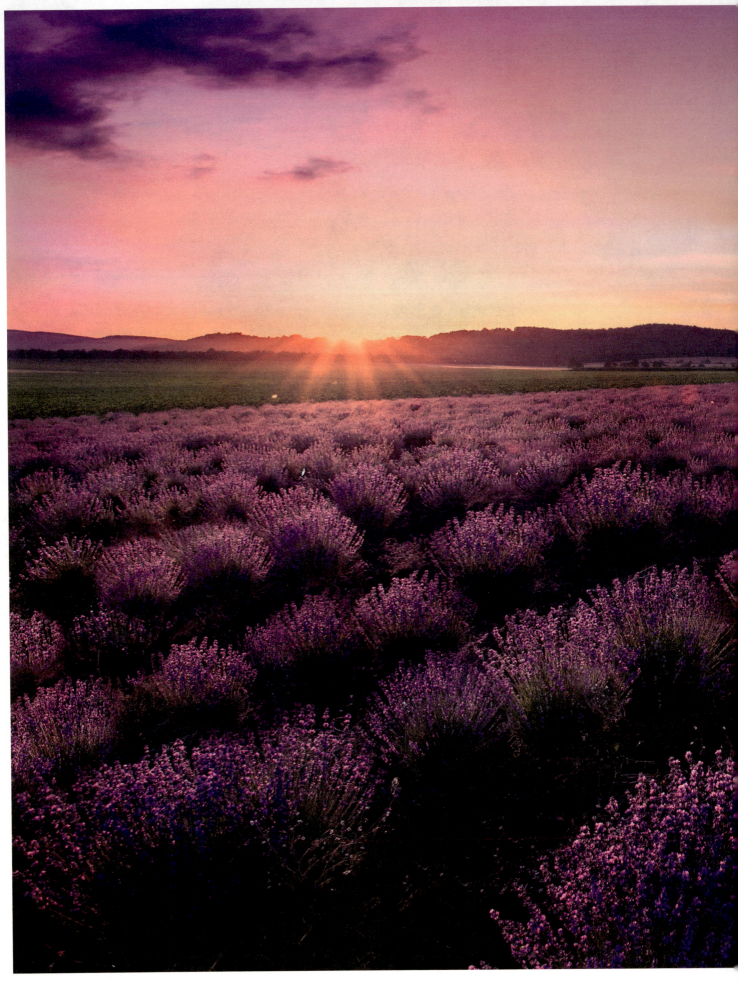

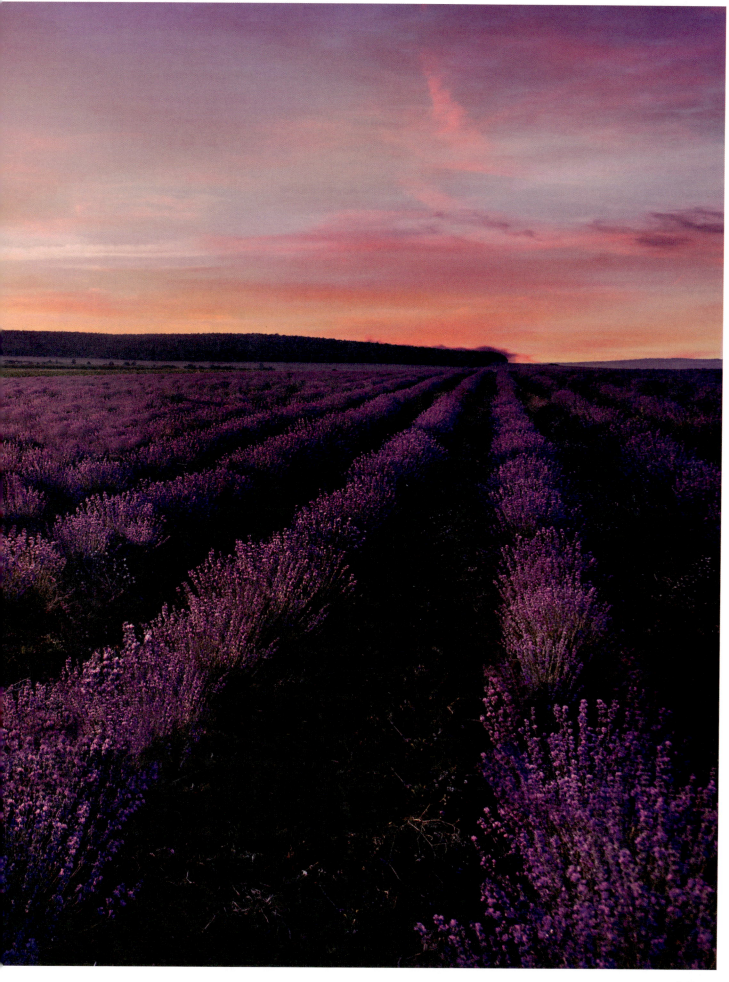

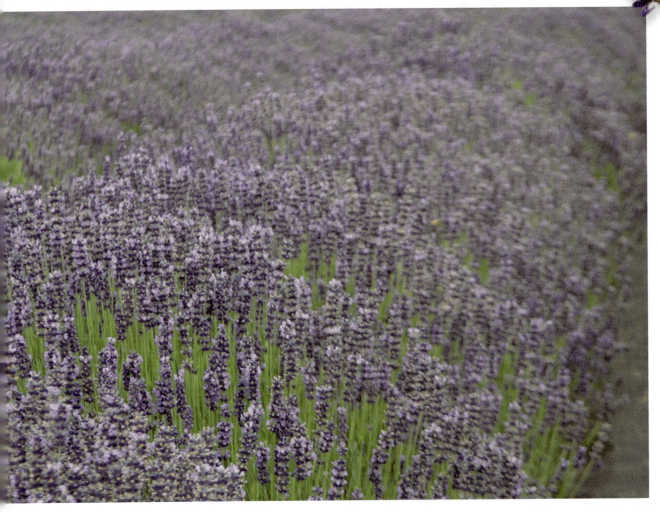

If you remember anything about growing lavender from this book, it would be to keep your plants "high and dry." It sounds like a line from an old western or some herbal folklore, but it is an easy way to remember that these drought-tolerant plants really do not like being wet. If you do not have a dry, sunny section in your yard, you may consider growing lavender in a container.

Lavender loves well-drained soil, lots of sunshine, and a slightly alkaline soil pH. It also needs to be pruned rather aggressively in the fall. Some growers also prune again in the spring to encourage growth and keep the plants looking neat and tidy. It is a valuable landscape plant if you live where there is threat of fire

danger or where you have wildlife. Deer don't really like lavender, and although they will sometimes nibble on the new green leaves, they mostly leave the plants alone. Lavender isn't fireproof, but it is a suggested plant for "firescaping," or landscaping with plants that will not burn down your home. Lavender is often one that is suggested since it can be grown near concrete, gravel paths, and patios.

Because lavender loves to be dry, well-drained soil is necessary. An easy way to test your soil is to dig a hole and fill it with water. If the water drains easily, then go ahead and plant your lavender. If, on the other hand the water is slow to drain or just sits in the hole, you are going to have to amend the soil with some hard bark, sand, or gravel. The need to keep the roots out of standing water is why you often see lavender planted on hillsides, raised beds, or elevated planting areas. If you visit a lavender farm, oftentimes the rows of lavender are planted on small mounds about six inches above the ground, which helps with drainage.

In addition to well-drained soil, lavender needs full sun. In fact, lavender loves full sun! Some varieties may grow in partial shade, however, if you plant the same variety in full sun, it will almost double in size. Before planting your lavender, really watch your yard and the amount of sunshine on each part. If your only spot is in the shade of a tree or large shrub, consider planting it in a container and placing it on a sunny deck or patio instead. Also think about what you are planting near your lavender. If nearby plants have different water or growing requirements, your garden will struggle. Plants that do well next to lavender include rosemary, basil, mint, and thyme. Lavender will also help plants that are dependent on pollination, as it attracts bees and other pollinators to your yard.

Lavender can thrive in most soil types, though it prefers a neutral or alkaline soil. If you wish to test your soil, purchase a simple kit at most garden stores. You will want to know your USDA Plant Hardiness Zone (see Page 23), as this is important when choosing which variety of lavender to plant. Lavender does not mind cold weather in the winter as long as it is dry. A good way to select plants is by talking to other gardeners and growers. Visit a local nursery or lavender farm, and don't be afraid to ask what varieties they are growing and with which ones they have had success. Oftentimes they will also tell you about ones that did not survive, even if they

Phytophthora Fungus

One disease that will kill your plants and could affect other garden plants is a fungus called *Phytophthora*. It's an algae in the soil that can cause root rot. You often cannot tell if your plants have been affected by it until it is too late. But if your plants are not thriving, especially in the spring and summer, you may want to have them tested. Most local county extension offices can help you, or point you in the right direction. If you have local lavender growers, you might also talk to them. If you are planting several lavender plants on a farm or as a border, this is another reason to purchase starts from a reputable nursery or farmer. To help avoid this root-rotting fungus, make sure your plants have good drainage. If you do end up with this fungus in your garden, pull out your plants and burn them; do not put them in your compost pile. Make sure to clean your garden tools really well to disinfect them to avoid spreading the disease.

were labeled for your hardiness zone. I visited one lavender farm in Kansas that had gone through several varieties over the years until they finally found the one that worked for them. They were happy to share their experiences in order to save other growers a few years of disappointment.

Few insects really bug lavender, which is why you often find lavender planted around gardens or outside of greenhouses. They act as a natural pest repellents for other garden plants, and also attract helpful bugs such as bees and ladybugs. The most common problem lavender growers experience is root rot or fungal infestations, which usually results from overwatering. Sometimes you may also purchase diseased plants. You can always take a few plants to your local agricultural extension service and have them tested and examined. This may

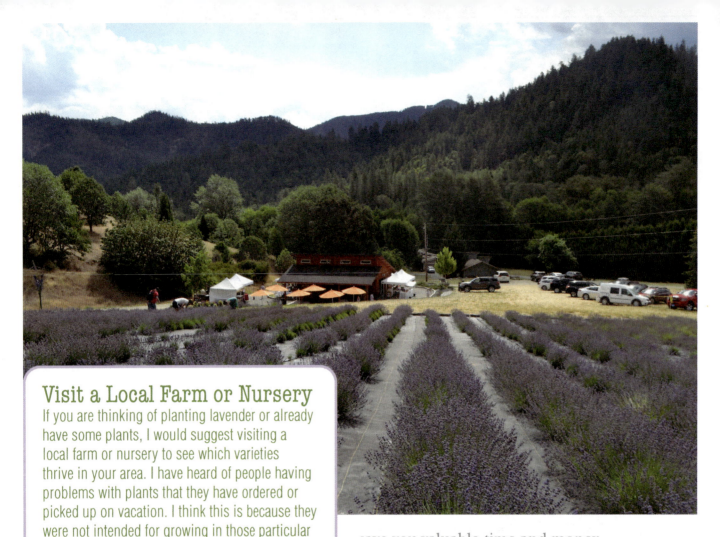

Visit a Local Farm or Nursery

If you are thinking of planting lavender or already have some plants, I would suggest visiting a local farm or nursery to see which varieties thrive in your area. I have heard of people having problems with plants that they have ordered or picked up on vacation. I think this is because they were not intended for growing in those particular regions or environments. Lavender farms are also really fun and interesting places to visit. They offer a wealth of information on lavender as well as other plants. They offer classes, activities, and events that can be enjoyed by all ages. My local farms offer dinners in the lavender fields during the summer. One lets you bring in your own plant material and learn to create essential oils and hydrosols. Many of them have animals such as miniature donkeys, goats, and geese. Some have tea shops where you can enjoy a cup of lavender tea or lemonade. Others have healthy activities such as yoga or walking a lavender labyrinth. In Michigan, there is a lavender farm so large you can see it from space! I also would not just visit these farms in the summer during the lavender bloom, which is the most popular time of year. I would also visit in the fall to see the plants after they have been pruned, getting ready for winter. The farms are usually still open and much more relaxed, and it also gives you another point of view of a working lavender farm.

save you valuable time and money. I feel it is always better to spend a bit more for a healthy plant from a reputable nursery or grower than to go with a "bargain" that may give you headaches down the road.

Starting Seeds and Cuttings

Having a good basic knowledge about how plants grow will help you become a successful gardener. There are several good books on gardening and information online so I am not going to try and cover everything; here are some basics to get you growing. Most plants start from seeds, and a few start from spores. Lavender can be started from both seeds and stem cuttings.

While starting lavender from seed is the most inexpensive way to start plants, it also takes the longest, as you may not see any blooms the first year as the young plants grow. If you have time and want a large number of plants for the least amount of money, seeds are the way to go. You just may not be able to find as large a variety from seeds, as most people prefer starting plants from starts or cuttings. If you do want to try starting plants from seeds, two varieties that work well are 'Lavender Lady' and 'Munstead'. You will need to plant them in seed-starting trays or flats. Lavender seeds are super-tiny, black, and very hard to see and handle. Sowing or sprinkling them on top of the soil then tamping them down is the easiest way to plant them and ensure success. (See "How to Build a Seed Tray" on Page 20.) Follow the instructions on the seed packet. Lavender seeds need at least three weeks of cold before being placed outside in full sun. Some growers use cold frames or old refrigerators to store their seed trays in before putting them in the sun. Use a light soil that drains well. Once the young plants have sprouted and have several leaves on them, plant them in the garden or containers. Make sure they are protected as they will grow very slowly the first year and can get knocked over or walked on by people and pets. The second year with full sun they will grow much better. I think it really takes about three years to get a decent size plant with blooms.

The easiest and most popular method for starting new lavender plants is with a stem cutting. Most growers prefer this method as they know that the cutting will be genetically identical to the original plant. The original plants are often called "mothers" and some gardens and farms are quite proud of them. I have seen mother plants proudly displayed at some farms whereas other farms hide them away to prevent people from taking cuttings and damaging the valuable plant. Garden etiquette requires us to always ask before taking a cutting of any plant. Gardeners, including lavender farmers, are some of the most generous people, if asked. (They can also get quite upset and may ask you to leave their grounds if they catch you cutting their plants.)

To create your own cuttings from your plants, choose a small branch and gently break it off. Most growers do this at the end of the growing season in late fall, though I have done it in the spring and had

Munstead Wood

Lavandula angustifolia 'Munstead' is a popular lavender cultivar and one of the easier varieties to start from seed. It is named after Munstead Wood, which is the house and garden of famous garden designer Gertrude Jekyll. Jekyll was a well-known English gardening writer and designer who lived from 1897 to 1932. She created more than 400 gardens and wrote more than 1,000 articles on the topic of garden design. Her home, Munstead Wood, is a popular tourism spot on the national register of historic parks and gardens in England. You will see many varieties of English lavender in the garden. It is located in Munstead Heath, Busbridge, on the border of the town of Godalming in Surrey, England.

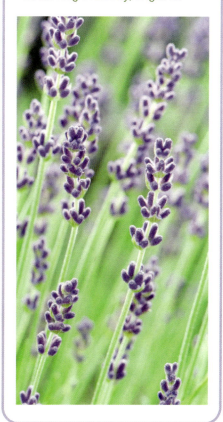

How to Build a Seed Tray

Most seed-starting trays sold in the stores are made of plastic. They are inexpensive, lightweight, and don't leak. One problem with plastic trays is that they do not breathe or allow for movement of air and moisture, so you can sometimes lose seeds to rot or mold. If you have ever had to carry the trays in and out of the house, you will notice they also are a bit flimsy. Wood trays have been used for years, well before the invention of plastic, and they make excellent seed-starting containers. Wood is naturally porous, so it provides better drainage and aeration for the plant roots. It's easy to reuse scrap pieces of wood leftover from other projects. With proper care, your wood trays should last several growing seasons, and can be used for starting any seeds. Here are the basic instructions; feel free to be creative and adapt to what you have on hand. You can also add drawer handles to each end to make your tray easier to carry. The scrap piece of wood is for tamping down seeds.

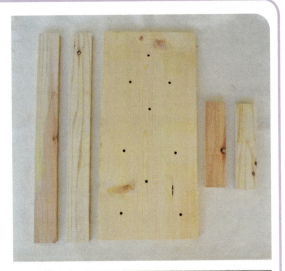

TOOLS AND MATERIALS FOR ONE TRAY:

Wood screws
Wood glue (optional)
Drill
Screwdriver
24-inch piece of wood 1x12 inches (1)
24-inch pieces of wood 1x2½ inches (2)
10-inch pieces of wood 1x2½ inches (2)
1 piece of scrap wood (about 9x7 inches)
1 to 3 recycled drawer handles

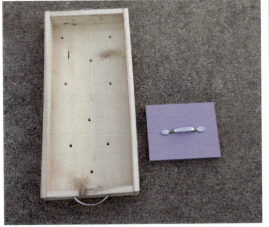

TO BUILD: Drill about 10 to 12 holes on the largest (24x12-inch) piece of wood. This is your tray bottom, so the holes help with drainage. Build a simple frame with the four 1x2½-inch pieces. Attach the bottom to the sides of the frame, using wood glue to hold everything in place. Let it all dry, then use a drill to insert the wood screws. Screw the drawer handles to the frame. Finally, attach an old drawer handle to your scrap piece of wood for tamping down seeds.

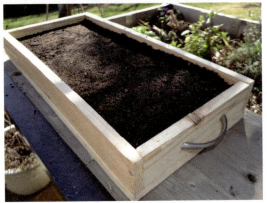

TO PLANT: Fill with damp seed-starting mix, and sprinkle with lavender seeds. Tamp down the mixture and add a bit more soil to cover. Spray the mixture. Place in a sunny spot, and periodically water or mist the soil with a spray bottle. When your starts have several leaves, you can gently move them to larger containers or garden beds.

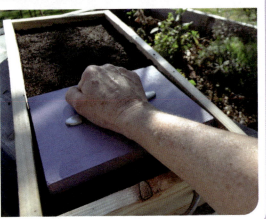

Propagation in Water

A quick method of propagating a lavender start is to place it in a jar of water as you would with mint. Cut a few healthy stems and remove the leaves from the lower section; place in the jar. Change the water every day and leave the jar in a well-lit northern- or eastern-facing window. In about 6 to 8 weeks you should see tiny roots begin to form. Then, plant your rooted cuttings in small pots full of clean potting soil. Keep the soil moist, but not too wet, and your new plants should be ready for transplant in a few months.

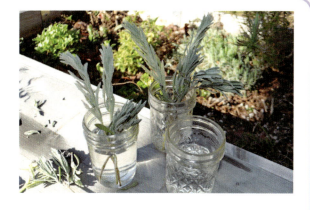

success. So experiment with your own plants. The length of your cutting should be about 6 inches. Use clippers, though I have heard it is better to break or tear the section off the main plant. Remove several of the lower leaves, halfway up the cutting.

Using a small stick or skewer, make a small hole in a pot filled with soil or in the ground, and place the cutting inside. Water your cutting and keep the soil moist, but not too wet, as the young start develops roots. This should take about six to eight weeks. You should notice it begin to green up and grow.

Some people like to use rooting hormone powder or liquid before planting their cuttings. I have done both and had about equal success.

I feel it really is the quality of the cutting that makes the difference. Also, I should note, not all of your cuttings will take. I often have some that just will not grow. This is why it is a good idea to start more cuttings than you will really need.

These cuttings are basically free plants, so having a few extra will ensure you end up with ones you can plant, sell, or give to friends.

Another way to source new lavender plants is to simply purchase them from a farm or good nursery. Usually these plants are a few years old, and you can instantly add them to your garden or yard and harvest blooms the first year.

Hardy vs. Tender Lavender

Lavender varieties are described as either hardy or tender. Read plant descriptions and know your USDA Plant Hardiness Zone (see map on Page 23) to determine the best varieties for your area. Some varieties can withstand a heavy frost and will come back year after year. Visit your local agriculture extension office; the agents are knowledgeable about the area's hardiness zones, soil testing, pests, diseases, and plant sources.

Doing a bit of homework is time well spent. I have made the mistake of buying the first lavenders I see at the home supply stores only to have them wilt and die after the first year. Knowing whether you have a hardy plant or a tender one will make all the difference, especially if you live in a cold weather zone.

Take the time to observe your yard, making sure to not plant them in a wet or shady spot. Lavender is also a drought-tolerant

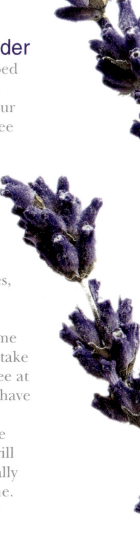

plant, so if you have an area of your yard where other plants have not survived, you may try lavender there. It is one of the plants used in "xeriscaping," a type of landscaping where the need for water is reduced or eliminated. Once established, lavender needs very little water to flourish.

Some people also use mulch around their plants such as small gravel or shells. You want something that will reduce weeds while not absorbing moisture. Avoid using fine bark that absorbs water and could cause fungus to grow.

Plan for mature plants. Don't plant young plants close together. Space them three to four feet apart; once established, your lavender plants will bloom and spread out. It is so much easier to prune and harvest your plants when you can work between them.

Hardy or Tender?

There are several varieties of lavender with different degrees of hardiness. Hardy lavenders are native to the Mediterranean and also called English lavenders. They are considered perennials, which means they will go dormant in the winter and bloom again in the spring. Some popular hardy lavender varieties include:

Old English (*Lavandula angustifolia*)
L. angustifolia 'Munstead'
L. angustifolia 'Folgate'
L. angustifolia 'Hidcote'
L. angustifolia 'Ellagance Pink'
L. intermedia 'Dutch'
L. intermedia 'Alba'
Woolly lavender (*L. lanata*)

Tender lavenders are native to Spain and southern France, also known as French lavenders. They are more sensitive to temperature and may not make it through a cold frost or winter. They need full sun and rich soil. Some popular varieties of tender lavenders are:

Spanish Lavender (*L. stoechas*)
French Lavender (*L. dentata*)
Green Lavender (*L. viridis*)
Sweet Lavender (*L. heterophylla*)

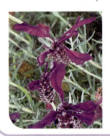 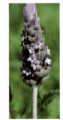 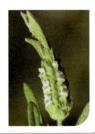

Growing Lavender In Containers

You can grow lavender in containers, but you will need large pots or containers since the roots like to spread out. You may start smaller plants in smaller containers, but you will need to transfer them. I know some people say not to plant lavender in a pot. I think this is because most people have the tendency to overwater them and let the roots sit in water, which will cause the plant to wither and even die. The best pots I have found are large terra cotta ones with good drainage. The material is porous, so it allows moisture to evaporate through the pot walls. I like to use pots for tender varieties of lavender. It allows me to move them close to the house or into the greenhouse during cold winter months. It also allows me to move them into full sun in the summer. I would not put other plants in with your lavender because they'll get squeezed out over time. Plus not every plant can go without watering like lavender can.

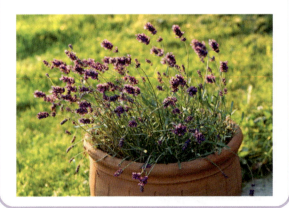

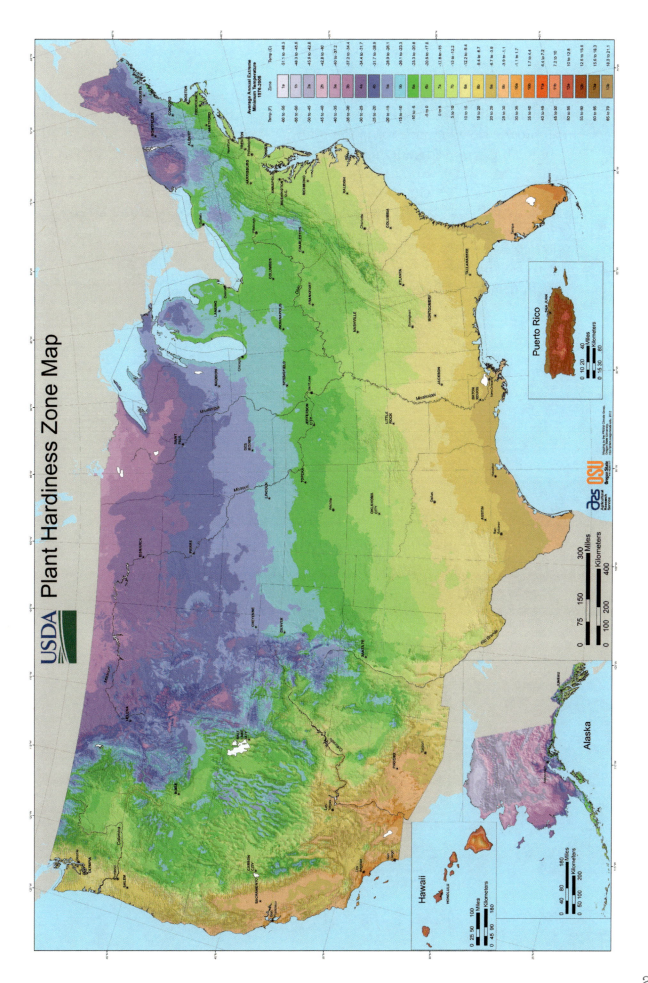

USDA Plant Hardiness Zone Map

Lavender is tolerant and not too picky about soil type as long as it is dry and drains well. If you wish to record your garden soil and keep track of how your plants do, use this chart.

SOIL TESTING RESULTS

Date	Location	pH results	Action taken

MY GARDEN DESIGN

Each Square = 1 Square Foot

SEED STARTING/GERMINATION RECORD

Seed Variety	Source of Seed	Date Planted	# of Days to Germination	Comments	Transplant Date (if started indoors)	Comments

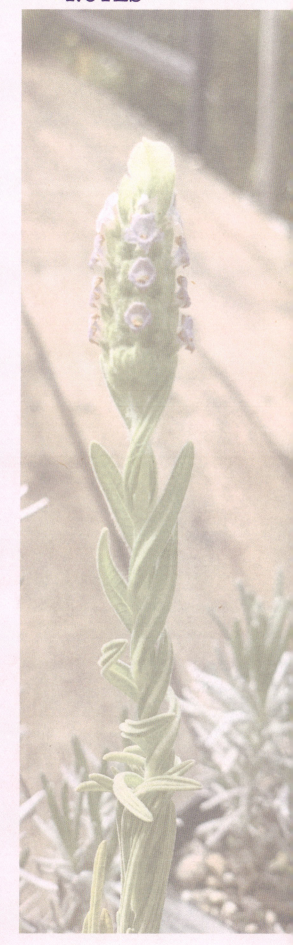

How to Use the Seed Starting Worksheet

Track your lavender seed varieties from one season to the next, and keep track of what works well for you and your garden (see opposite page).

1. In the first column, note the lavender variety.
2. Note the source of your seeds.
3. Note the date you planted your seeds.
4. Note how many seeds you planted so you can keep track of your germination rate.
5. Write comments on successes or things you learned.
6. Note the date you transplanted your young plants if started in seed trays.
7. Make comments on transplanting; What worked well? What could be improved?

How to Use the Lavender Starts Worksheet

On the next page, track your lavender cuttings and varieties from one season to the next, and keep track of what works well for you.

1. In the first column, note the lavender variety.
2. List the source of your cutting.
3. Note the date you planted your cuttings and how many.
4. Did you use a rooting hormone? If so, note the name and company.
5. Note how many cuttings you planted took root, so you can keep track of your success rate.
6. Note comments on success or things you learned.
7. When did you transplant your young plants if started in starter pots?
8. Note comments on transplanting; what worked well, what can be improved.

LAVENDER STARTS RECORD

Mother Plant or Lavender Variety	Source	Date Planted	Rooting Hormone Used? Yes/No	# of Days to Root	Comments	Transplant Date	Comments

Parts of the Lavender Plant

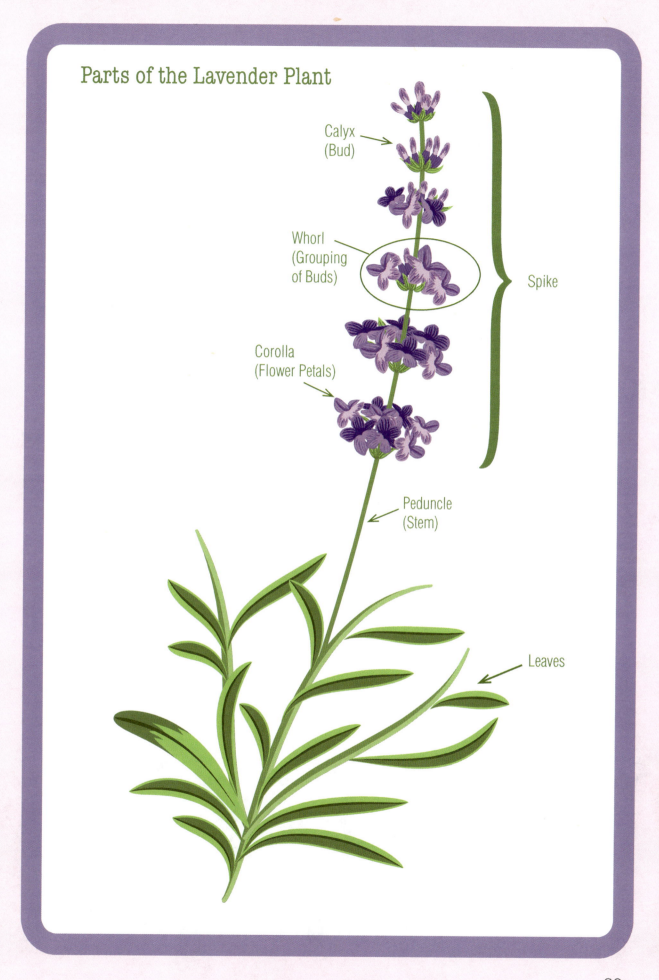

Calyx (Bud)

Whorl (Grouping of Buds)

Corolla (Flower Petals)

Spike

Peduncle (Stem)

Leaves

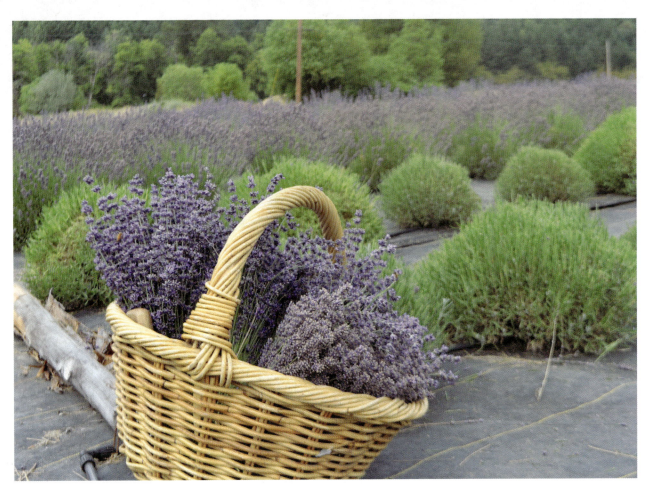

Harvesting Lavender

Harvesting and pruning your lavender encourages more growth, giving you more flowers the next year. It also keeps your plants tidy so they look better in your yard and garden.

The question of when to harvest your lavender depends on what type you are growing and what you intend to use it for. If you grow it for culinary use, harvest when the buds are just emerging and tight, and still full of natural oils. For floral bouquets, about a third of the buds should be open and still tight enough to remain on the stem.

For sachets and loose dried buds, wait a bit longer, as it does not matter if your flowers are attached to the stems.

Lavender is easy to harvest. Remember to leave a few leaves (about four or six sets) to remain on each stem to allow the plant to regrow. If you cut into the woody stems, they may not return. (See lavender pruning tips on Page 37.)

This is my favorite time of the growing season and when I really feel like a "lavender farmer."

I like to use my lavender for creating bath and body-care products and for filling simple sachets. So I am not as concerned about the look of the buds. Plus, I am a beekeeper and most of my lavender is close to my beehive, so I like to leave the flowers for the bees as long as I can.

When it is time to harvest my flower buds, I lay a large cotton tablecloth or sheet on the ground. As I cut the lavender, I pile it on the cloth. Some people like to tie their lavender in bundles, which works too, and I will get to that method. For me, it's all about cutting and piling.

I wrap my lavender in the tablecloth or sheet, and move it to a table set up on my patio. I keep the plant material out

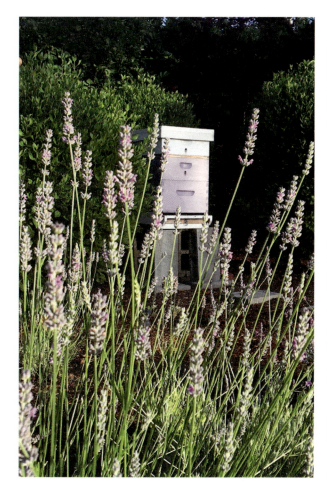
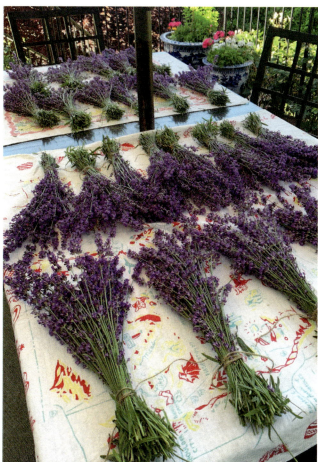

of direct sunlight, leaving it on the table and turning it each time I walk by (two or three times a day).

Once the lavender has dried, I pat or thrash the stems, allowing the lavender buds to fall off. Then I scoop up the buds and place them in large bowls or trays. I continue this method until all the buds are off the stems. I save the stems for making fire starters (see Page 97), or for use in pet beds. The really long ones work well for natural skewers and toothpicks for serving food.

That is my method, and I sometimes have several tables full. My husband once joked that most people want more bathrooms in their homes, whereas we need more dining rooms so I can fill the tables with lavender. If it is really windy or there's bad weather, I often move my harvest indoors for drying.

If you visit a lavender farm or talk to other growers, you will hear a variety of methods. The most common one is to cut your lavender into small bundles using a tool that looks like a small sickle or curved knife. Small handheld pruning shears work too.

Gather your lavender stems into small bunches about 2 inches in diameter. You do not want your bunches too large, as they could mold or mildew in the center without proper airflow. If you want a really large bunch, combine your smaller ones once dried.

Use a rubber band to secure the lavender, which will contract as the bunches dry to keep them tidy. If you tie your bunches with garden twine; make sure it is nice and tight as the bundles will get smaller as they dry.

For drying, use my method of laying the bunches on a tabletop as I do; turn them a few times during the day. You can also hang them flower-side down (this keeps the stems nice and straight). The hanging method works especially well if you are using your lavender in dried flower

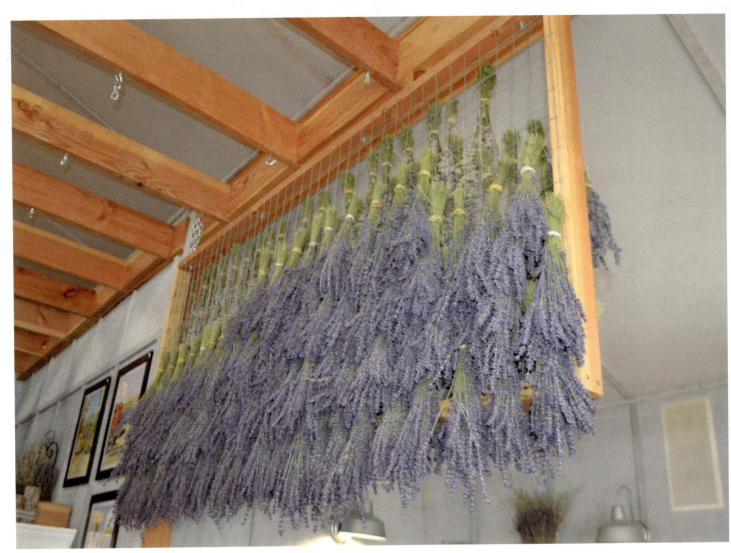

arrangements. Hang them from laundry racks, chains, or even frames made with farm fencing. Straighten a paper clip to make a small hook, and arrange your bundles on these racks.

I have heard of people using food dehydrators or their ovens to dry lavender. I have not tried this as I feel the air drying method works the best and gives me the best results. It really does not take that long, especially in hot weather.

Once I am sure it is dry, I store my lavender in glass jars. To keep the color, store the jars in a dry, dark spot. You can purchase special amber or UV-filtering jars. Storing them in a cupboard works best for me.

After your lavender bunches are dried, if you wish to harvest the buds, you can simply massage them over a large bowl or tray, and they will drop off the stem.

Some people also strain their buds with a bit of screen to remove any bits of stem or leaves. I don't usually bother with this step as I don't mind a few "extras" in my buds. I have also seen de-budding machines for purchase. They have either soft brushes or shakers in which to load the bundles, and the machines then remove the buds, dumping the buds into a bucket. They are interesting machines to watch, though they are oftentimes an expensive purchase for the average grower. At the most recent U.S. lavender conference I attended, they had one of these huge de-budding machines in the lobby. It was definitely a conversation piece and every night several people would gather around to watch the dried buds being threshed and spit out into a bucket. It also made the whole hotel smell amazing, and I am sure everyone slept really well that night.

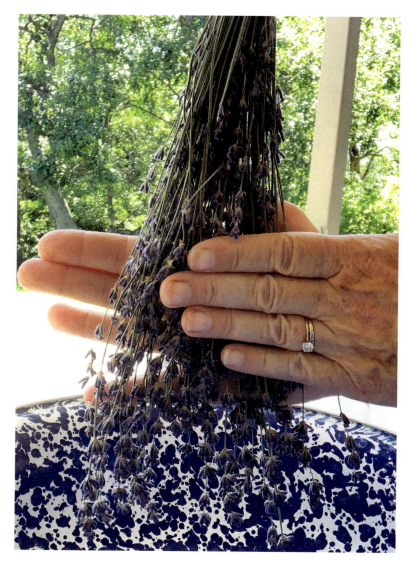

Lavender Essential Oil

Lavender oil is a common and popular essential oil found in almost every natural food store. It is used in aromatherapy, body-care products, and as a useful household product. You can make your own oils at home using a simple still. While it takes a lot of plant material to produce a small amount of oil, many farmers and growers find this to be a rewarding process. They feel they capture the pure essence of their plants.

If you do not have your own still or don't want to purchase one your first year of growing, some farms will let you use theirs. In my area, one of the farms will allow you, for a fee, to bring your plant material and use their still. It might be worth taking a class in distilling plant material, as the process is the same.

Distilling plant oils means basically steaming them and then capturing the steam that contains the plant oils. For lavender, it takes about 3 pounds of plant material to create three teaspoons of oil. For this

Harvesting Tips

Here are a few tips for a successful lavender harvest.

• Pick the mature stems early in the morning, just after the dew has had a chance to dry. This will give you stems full of natural oils and with a nice fragrance.

• Do not pick your lavender if it is wet, as it will take longer to dry and you could end up with mold or mildew.

• The stems should be cut where they meet the leaves. Allow some leaves to remain so the plant will continue to grow.

• After harvesting, feed your plants with a little lime or compost, and you may get a second bloom.

• Prune your plants in the fall to get them ready for winter. Some growers trim the plants again in the spring to encourage new growth.

• Use clean tools; you do not want to introduce any diseases or fungus. This is true for any and all your garden plants.

• Store your dried lavender in a well-ventilated, dry, dark spot. Some lavender farms have drying barns that are fun to tour and smell amazing.

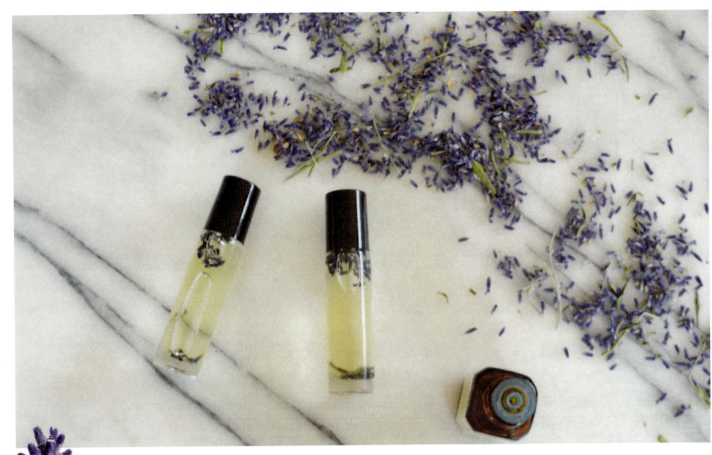

reason many people will often create infused oils and skip the distilling process. (Especially if you only have a few plants.)

The process of capturing the oil is called "steam distillation," or simply "distillation." It basically involves filling a pot or a still with water and plant material. If you are distilling lavender, you will want to cut your flowers when they have bloomed and are full of oil. You want to really fill your pot or still with the flower heads. Heating the water will cause steam to pass through the lavender and release all the natural essential oils. The steam then passes through a condenser, cooling down, and becoming a liquid called a hydrosol. You will see a thin layer of oil floating on top of the cooled steam. The amount of oil you will see depends on a couple factors: the variety of lavender harvested and when the lavender was harvested. The most common variety of lavender used in oil production is 'Grosso' lavender. English lavender is also used. The lavender oil is gently removed from the hydrosol using a pipette or eyedropper. Personally, I believe the hydrosol is just as valuable as lavender oil. It has a lovely scent and is easily used to create body-care products. It can be used alone as a body spray or linen spray.

I suggest creating a makeshift still on your stovetop using kitchen equipment. Some systems use the microwave; while I've tested one of these, and it worked, the price tag, time spent, and amount of oil produced, I feel, wasn't worth it. The system might work for farms to test their plant oils quickly; for the average gardener, it is perhaps too involved for the few drops of essential oil produced.

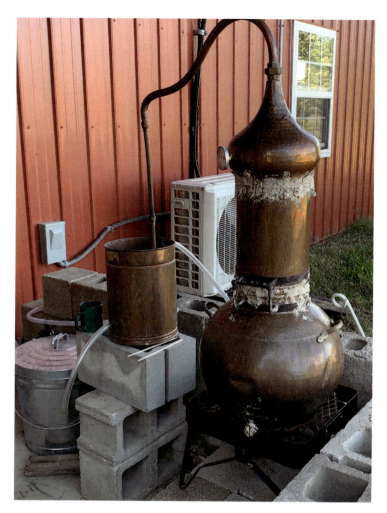

Oil Distillation Process

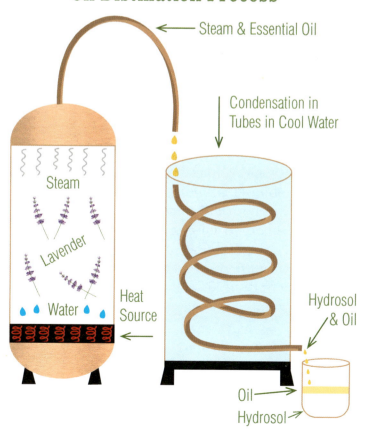

Steam & Essential Oil

Condensation in
Tubes in Cool Water

Steam

Lavender

Water

Heat
Source

Hydrosol
& Oil

Oil

Hydrosol

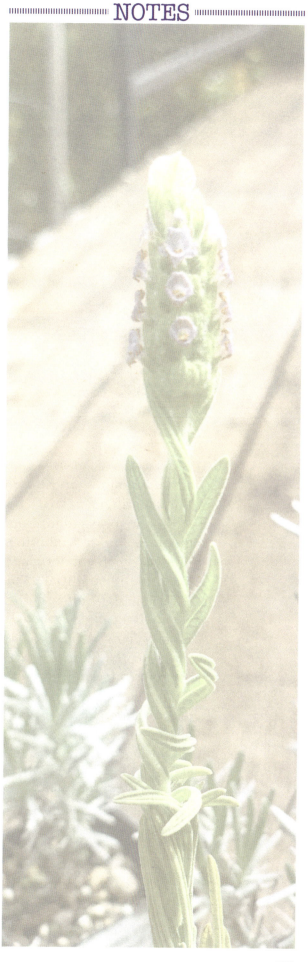

MY FAVORITE LAVENDERS

Name	Bloom Color	Size	Uses	# of Blooms	Comments

How to Prune Your Lavender

One of the most important things you can do to keep your plants looking their best and producing lots of flowers is to prune them in the fall. Some growers prune their plants in the spring, too.

It is a simple process, and your plants will love it!

If you don't trim your plants, they may show signs of stress and branch out in all sorts of ways, and you won't get as many blooms the following year.

When you purchase new plants, or young plants bloom for the first time, cut off all the blooms. I know this is difficult to do. It will help give your plant the energy it needs to grow, and, in the long run, you will end up with a healthier plant and more blooms.

Lavender is a fast-growing plant, oftentimes doubling in size from spring to fall.

In the fall, after you have harvested your last flowers, it is time for a good pruning.

Prune your plants into a ball shape. Don't be afraid to really cut your plants back. You want to train them into a nice compact shape, or else they will become leggy and woody, and you could even lose your plants or part of them.

Keeping them trimmed will keep them healthy, and you will be able to enjoy your plants for many years.

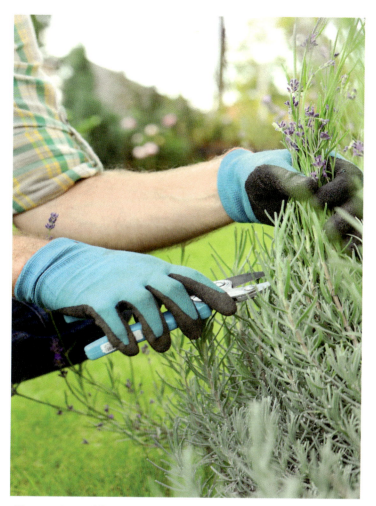

Pruning Extends the Life of Plants

Prune in fall and spring after flowering. Prune all shoots by at least a third.

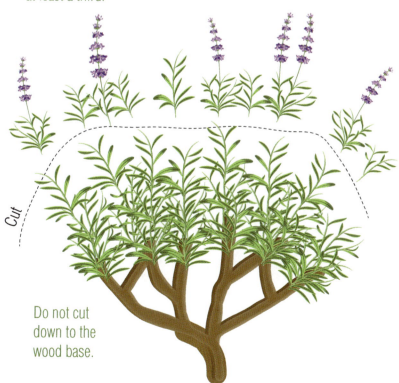

Cut

Do not cut down to the wood base.

GROWING LESSONS LEARNED

Date	Location	Best Variety	Least Productive Variety	Pest and Disease Problems and Solutions That Worked	Notes on Weather	Ideas for Crop Improvements	Questions to Research

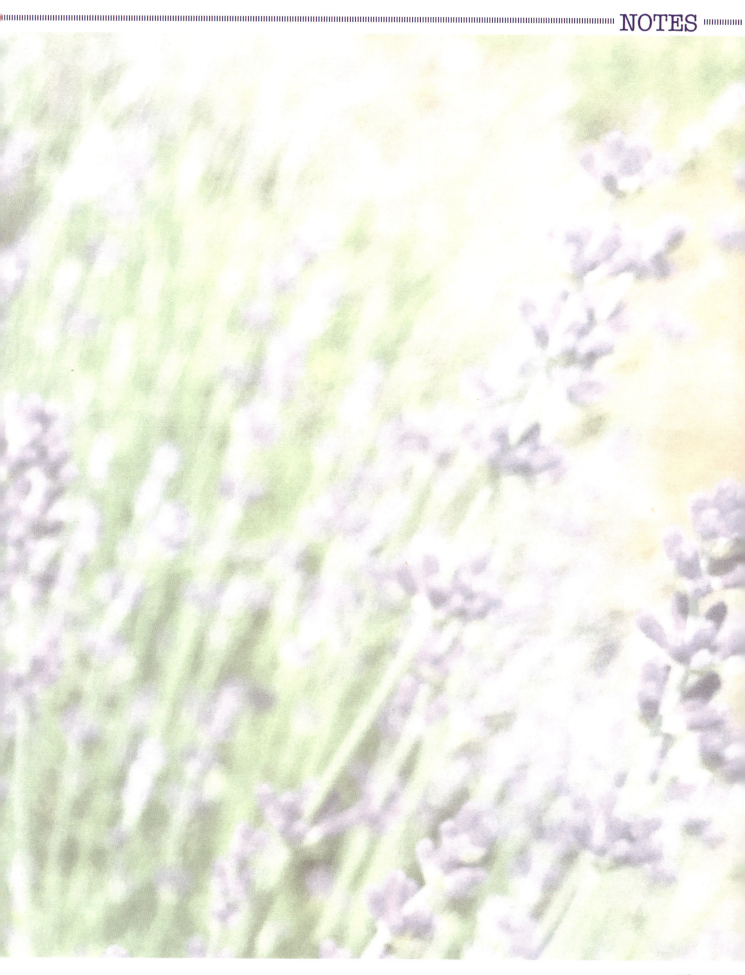

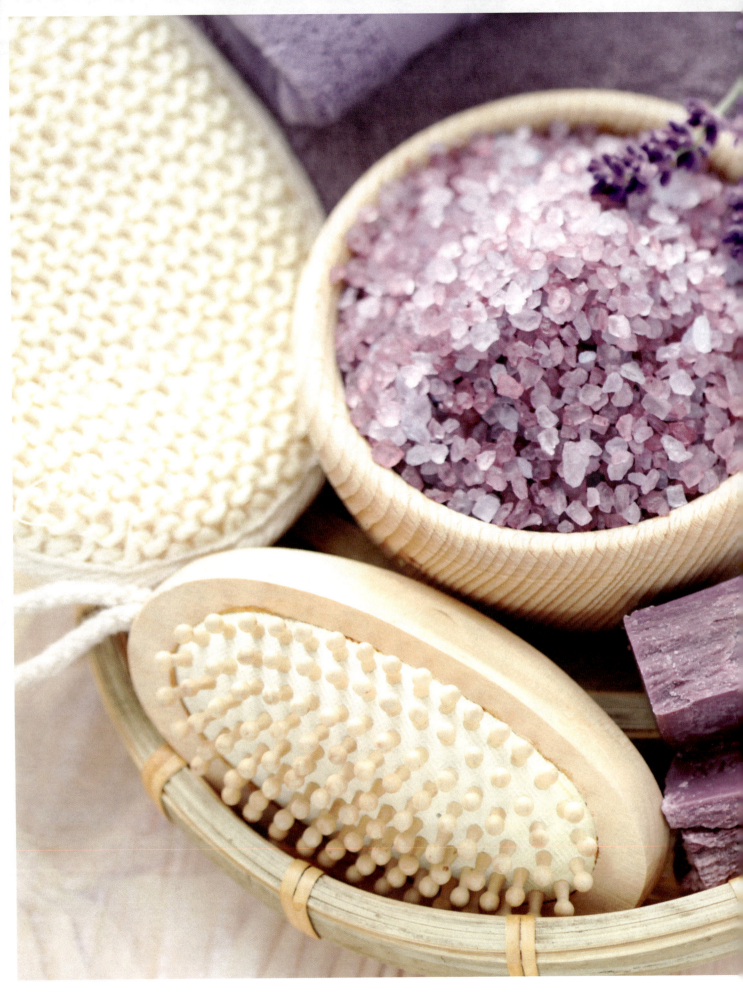

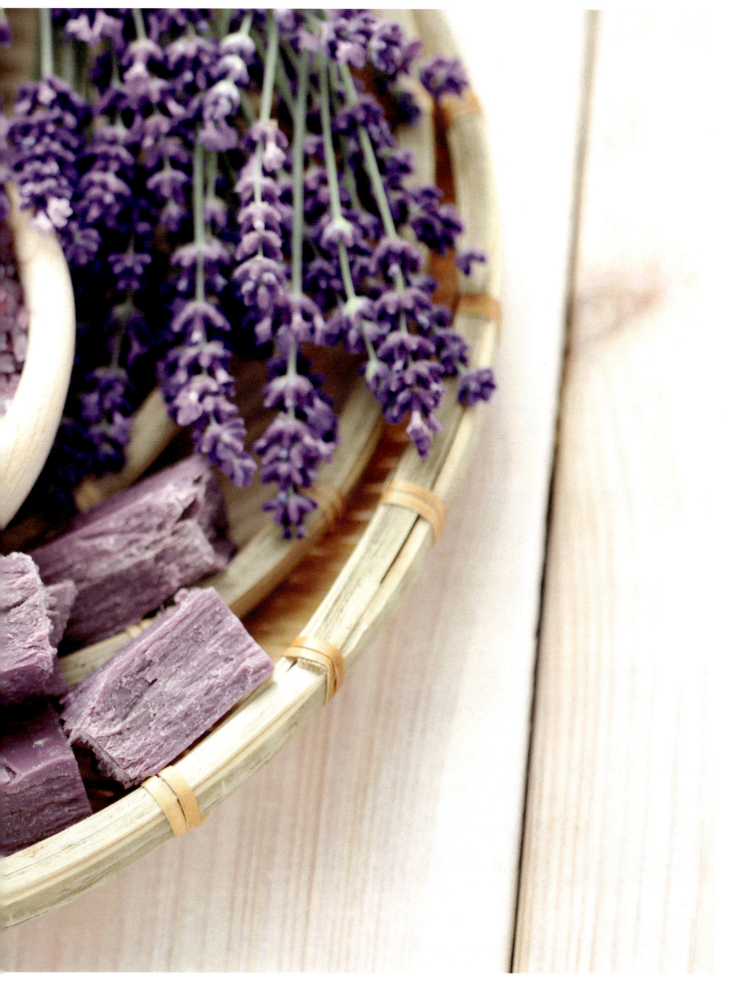

Chapter 2: Beauty & Lavender

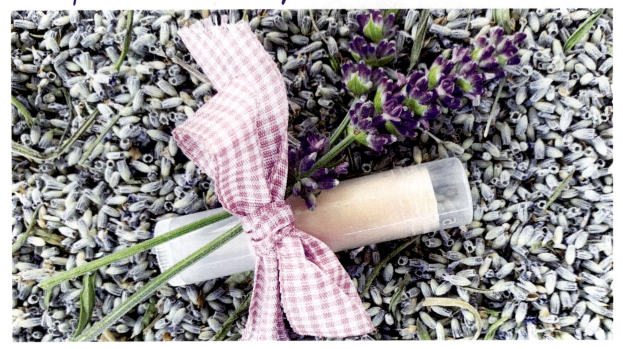

The smell of lavender is one of my earliest childhood memories. My grandmother made several of her own creams, bath products, and home remedies, and she also saved all the free product samples for me when I visited. She was particularly fond of gardenia, rose, and lavender. They all found a place on her bathroom shelf, though it was lavender that took up the most space. I would take long bubble baths at her house and use up all of her English lavender bath tablets. Whenever I returned to her house, I'd find a new box of tablets had appeared in the cupboard. While she had so many different soaps and lotions, I remember those tablets the best. It was not until later in life that I truly understood how the scent of lavender could be used to calm the body and the mind.

Today, lavender is a key ingredient in almost every type of body-care product on the market, from facial toners to bath products. The easily recognizable scent is both calming and cleansing, and perfect for all skin types. Lavender is one of the most fragrant and versatile herbs, especially when it comes to body-care products. Lavender also has anti-bacterial and anti-inflammatory properties. If you have a troubled complexion, use lavender to calm and cleanse it. As a hair-care product, lavender will deeply cleanse your scalp. Healthy hair results from a healthy scalp.

Lavender and lavender essential oil are useful in boosting hair growth and healing your skin. Just a dab of lavender oil on a small cut, scrape, or burn will help you heal. My husband carries a small roller bottle filled with lavender oil in his backpack and uses it as a skin "cure-all" when he travels. The scent also helps him sleep. If you get a bad sunburn, a strong infusion of lavender oil or lavender tea can help with some of the discomfort. Simply spray it on your scorched skin, or soak cotton fabric in a lavender solution and apply to your skin.

Here are some of my favorite DIY beauty recipes and treatments using this fragrant and skin-soothing plant.

Lavender Infusions

Because of its strong, clean scent and flavor, lavender infuses easily and quickly with other natural products, sometimes in a matter of hours. Natural oils, honey, sugar, salt, butter, vinegar, and alcohols all can be scented and flavored with fresh or dried lavender buds and leaves.

When making infused oils, use only dried plant material; added moisture from fresh plants could cause bacteria to grow in your products. For all other infusions, fresh or dried lavender will work. Just remember a simple rule of thumb: Dried lavender has twice the strength of fresh plants, so adjust the amount you use accordingly for each recipe.

Create simple infusions by adding lavender to your favorite ingredient. For example, to create a lavender sugar, place some lavender into your sugar jar, wait a few days, and then sample the mixture; you will detect notes of lavender. You can then strain your sugar and use it in your favorite recipe, or sprinkle it on fresh fruit. If you desire a stronger mixture, either add more lavender, or wait a few more days for it to infuse.

Here are a few sample proportions for various infusions. Keep track of your own infusions on the workbook page (on Page 44), and experiment with other herbs and ingredients to make your own unique combinations.

• **Honey:** Add 1 teaspoon dried lavender to ½ cup raw honey. Gently warm, then let the mixture sit for a few days.

• **Natural Oil:** Add 1 tablespoon dried lavender buds to 1 cup almond, grapeseed, sunflower, or coconut oil. Let sit for a week, then strain. For coconut oil, you will want to melt it before adding the lavender buds.

• **Sugar and Salt:** Add 1 teaspoon lavender buds to 1 cup sugar or salt. Let sit for one week to infuse. If you do not want lavender bits in your mixture, place the buds inside a piece of cheesecloth or muslin within your sugar or salt bowl.

• **Vinegar:** Lavender Vinegar is super easy to make and creates a beautiful shade of pink when used with white vinegar. Add 1 teaspoon dried lavender to 1 cup vinegar. See Page 50 for Lavender Vinegar Hair Rinse.

• **Alcohol:** Lavender infuses quickly into alcohol, almost within hours. Add 1 teaspoon dried lavender to 1 cup gin, vodka, or tequila.

Lavender Oil Health Benefits

Antiseptic: Lavender's germ-fighting properties keep your skin clean and feeling fresh.

Anti-inflammatory: Lavender has skin-soothing properties.

Reduces anxiety: Lavender's aroma has been shown to reduce anxiety and depression.

Aids sleep: This is probably the most well-known use of lavender. People often place some dried buds under their pillow or scent their sheets with lavender water sprays.

Treats skin issues: Lavender's anti-bacterial properties work well in healing salves and lotions for minor scrapes.

Relieves headaches: People who suffer from migraine headaches often use scented lavender oil as a remedy. Simply massaging a few drops on your temples will help your body and mind relax.

Calms sunburns: A strong infusion or tea made with lavender buds can help alleviate some of the discomfort from a painful sunburn.

MY LAVENDER INFUSIONS

Name	Infusion Type	Amount of Infusion Ingredient	Amount of Lavender	Other Ingredients	Results	How I Used It

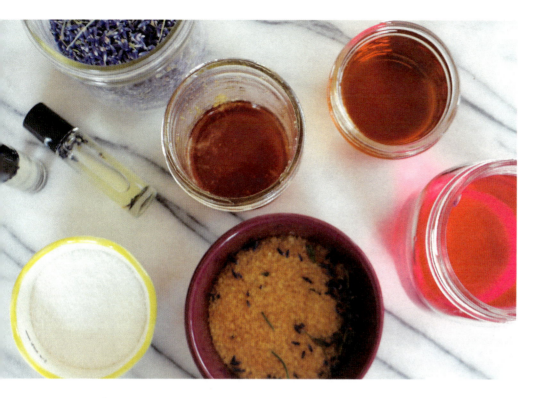

Creating Your Own Body-Care Products

The recipes in this section are easy to create at home using common kitchen equipment and ingredients such as natural cooking oils, herbal teas, and honey. The key ingredient is, of course, lavender. For the following recipes, preservatives are unnecessary, either because the ingredients act as a natural preservative, or the recipe yields enough for only one application. If you are sensitive to a known ingredient, feel free to use a substitute. For example, if you do not care for almond oil, or you have an allergy to it, try using light sesame or olive oil in its place. If you have a known food allergy, chances are you will also be allergic to a cosmetic product with that same ingredient.

Always take care when using any new products, whether homemade or commercial. To spot-test your skin, add a small amount of the new product to the skin on the inside of your arm, or the back of your leg, and wait 24 hours. If there is no reaction, it is probably safe to proceed with its use. If you are extremely sensitive, it is always best to consult your physician before using any new product or treatment. Remember, you are the manufacturer of these products and quality control is your responsibility. Always work with clean equipment and pure ingredients.

Creating your own body-care products is extremely satisfying and fun, and combines the best aspects of crafting and cooking. Of course, the end products make you feel so good. They also make welcome gifts for friends and family.

Basic Care and Storage Guidelines

• Always store your products in clean jars and bottles.

• Keep your fingers out of the container as much as possible, and always wash your hands before handling cosmetics. When you dip your fingers into the containers, you can introduce foreign germs and materials. Use cotton balls, cotton swabs, or a small spoon, whenever possible, or pour your beauty products onto your clean hands.

• Store your products in a cool, dark, dry place, as heat and light can sometimes alter the composition of your products. Amber-colored UV-blocking jars work best.

• If the products separate, simply stir the mixture thoroughly or re-blend.

• If a product develops a foul odor, throw it out. Once a product has gone bad, there is no way to recover it. You will be safer making a new batch.

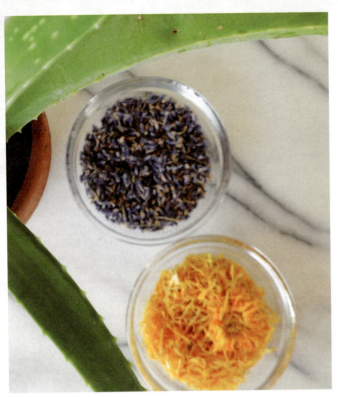

Massage Oil Herbs to Try

STIMULATING HERBS

Rosemary: Relieves apathy and boosts memory function

Oregano: Boosts circulation

Mint: Energizes and increases your metabolism

RELAXING HERBS

Chamomile: Relaxes the body and helps you sleep soundly

Lavender: Soothes and calms; also useful in curing headaches

Basil: Calms the nerves and relieves stress

Lavender-Calendula Gel

This gel is an excellent skin soother, and the sweet scent of calendula flowers (also known as pot marigolds) complements lavender well. In addition to the antiseptic properties of both calendula and lavender, lavender naturally heals skin irritations, burns, and insect stings with its calming quality. **Yield: 4 ounces**

½ cup aloe vera gel

1 tablespoon dried lavender buds or
   2 tablespoons fresh lavender buds

1 tablespoon dried calendula petals or
   2 tablespoons fresh calendula petals

Mix together the aloe vera gel, lavender buds, and calendula petals in an ovenproof glass container.

Heat the mixture gently, until very hot but not boiling. You can do this by placing the container in a water bath on the stovetop.

Let the mixture cool completely and sit for 24 hours. Strain out all of the flower petals and solids, and pour into a clean container.

To use: Massage into clean skin, or use on minor cuts, scrapes, and bites.

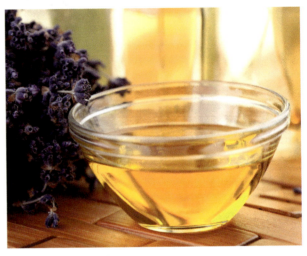

Relaxing Lavender Massage Oil

Lavender and dried herbs are perfect for making scented massage oils. Use this recipe as a bath oil, or make a welcome gift by placing a sprig of dried lavender inside a gift bottle. When infusing natural oils with lavender or any herb, only use dried plant material rather than introduce moisture that could cause bacteria to grow. I like to use lighter oils that absorb easily into the skin, such as grapeseed or jojoba oils. Feel free to use oils you enjoy. **Yield: 4 ounces**

½ cup grapeseed, jojoba, almond, or
   light sesame oil

1 tablespoon dried lavender

2 to 3 drops lavender essential oil
   (optional)

Mix together the oil and lavender. Heat gently on the stovetop in a water bath;

Roll-On Herb Combinations

If you want to experiment with other scents and create your own custom perfume blends, here are a few herbs to add to your roller bottle.

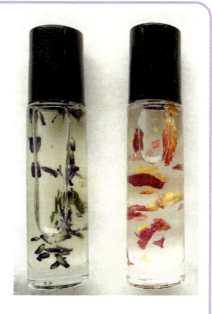

Relaxing: lavender, chamomile, and cinnamon
Energizing: lavender, dried citrus peel, and mint
Refreshing: lavender, eucalyptus, and cedar

Use only dried plant material when making scented oils. Vitamin E oil will act as a natural preservative and make your products last longer.

do not boil. Cool the mixture and let it sit overnight. The longer it sits, the stronger the scent will be. Strain out any solids, and pour into a clean bottle with a tight-fitting lid or cork stopper.

To use: Massage into your skin.

Note: You may also add other dried herbs or combinations of herbs to create your own unique oil blend. (See "Massage Oil Herbs to Try," Page 46.)

Roll-on Lavender Oil

I like to fill roller bottles with my favorite natural oil blends such as jojoba, almond, and avocado, and add dried lavender buds. You can add other dried herbs and a few drops of lavender essential oil. These make for on-the-go aromatherapy applicators, and are perfect for tucking inside pockets and totes. They also can be used on small cuts and scrapes. My husband keeps one in his backpack for just this reason.

Maybe you have a roller bottle that you can repurpose from home. You can also find them at natural food stores. **Yield: ½ to 1 ounce, depending on bottle size**

> 1 to 2 teaspoons almond, jojoba, argan, avocado, olive, or grapeseed oil
> ¼ teaspoon dried lavender buds
> 1 to 2 drops lavender essential oil
> 1-ounce glass roller bottle

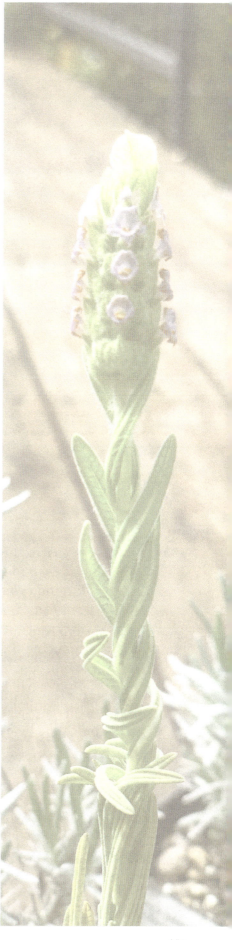

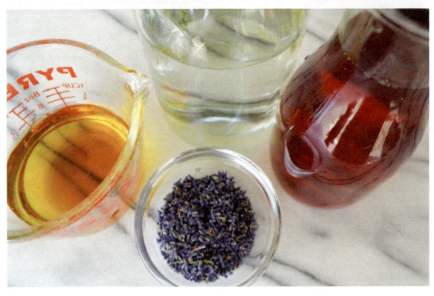

Fill the bottle with oil and add the dried herbs and essential oil. Let the bottle sit for a few days. If you would like a stronger scent, strain and repeat with more lavender and essential oil. If you feel the scent is too strong, strain and add more oil.

To use: Apply oil by rolling it over your wrist, neck, or inner elbow.

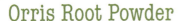

Orris Root Powder

The root of the white iris *(Iris florentina)* is used as a fixative in perfumes and powders. The dried root has a light scent of violet and originated in ancient Greece and Rome. Natural food stores carry this powder in their bulk bins. It is also very popular with those who make their own potpourris, so you may also find it where dried herbs and flowers are sold.

Lavender Dry Perfume

Dry perfumes are similar to sachets. Nefertiti, queen of Egypt during the 18th dynasty, always carried her personal scent with her in a small pouch attached at her waist. Dry perfumes have more intense aromas than powders, and are used to scent the skin and hair. **Yield: 1 ounce**

> 1 teaspoon orris root powder
> 1 tablespoon dried lavender buds
> 1 tablespoon cornstarch
> 2 drops lavender essential oil

Mix all ingredients together. Place the mixture in a food processor, blender, or coffee grinder and process until a smooth powder is achieved. (Use a mortar and pestle if you wish to grind the powder by hand.)
Place in a clean container with a tight-fitting lid.

To apply: Rub a small amount of this scented powder on your skin where you would apply liquid perfume or cologne.

Lavender Skin Freshener

Lavender essential oil comes from fresh lavender flowers and is well-known for its antiseptic (germ-killing) properties. You can learn to distill your own oil, or easily purchase it from a local farm or natural food store. (See more about lavender oil production on Page 32.) This recipe may be used on the face, or splashed on all over the body after a shower or bath.
Yield: 2 ounces

> 3 tablespoons purified water
> 2 tablespoons witch hazel
> 2 to 3 drops lavender essential oil
> ½ teaspoon vegetable glycerin
>   or honey

Mix all of the ingredients together. Pour into a clean bottle with a tight-fitting lid.

To apply: Apply to face or body with a clean cloth.

Lavender Shampoo

Adding herbs to a basic shampoo recipe can bring out natural highlights. In the case of lavender, it will enhance your natural

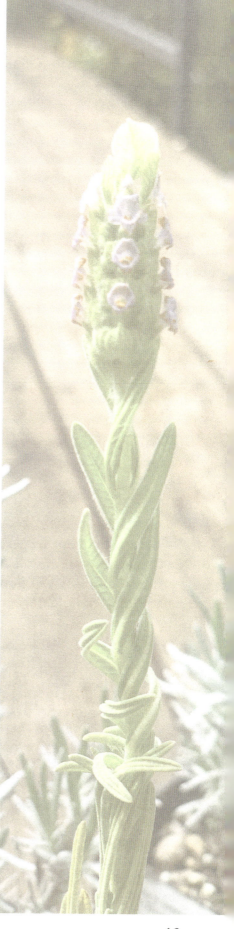
Borax Powder

Borax is a natural salt found on alkaline lake shores such as in California's Death Valley. It is used as a water softener, preservative, and texturizer. As a mild alkali, it gently cleanses without drying the skin. Borax powder can be found in the detergent section of the grocery store. Make sure you purchase products made from 100 percent borax.

hair color and may also have a darkening effect over time, as rosemary does. Homemade or all-natural shampoos also have less of a foaming effect, which may take time to get used to. They clean your scalp and hair just as well, although you may not have that full-head-of-suds effect that you are used to. I like to use castile soap when making this recipe; feel free to experiment with your own favorite liquid soap or natural shampoo. **Yield: 8 ounces**

½ **cup water**
2 **tablespoons dried lavender buds**
½ **cup liquid castile soap**
2 **tablespoons vegetable glycerin**

To use: Mix together the water and dried lavender; heat gently to make a strong tea. Let the mixture steep for at least 20 minutes. Strain out the solids, and add the soap and glycerin to the mixture. Stir well gently until completely blended. Pour the shampoo into a clean squeeze bottle or empty shampoo bottle. Let the mixture sit overnight to thicken.

To use: Shampoo as you would normally, and rinse well.

Lavender Leaf Shampoo Powder

Lavender leaves give the hair luster and shine. This shampoo powder is especially convenient when traveling or backpacking because it is so light and compact. Just add water when using in the shower or bath. For extra highlighting and a stronger scent, add some small dried lavender buds to the mixture, or a few drops of lavender essential oil. You can find lavender bud powder at some natural food stores, or easily make your own using a coffee or spice grinder. **Yield: 4 ounces**

½ **cup finely grated castile soap**
2 **teaspoons borax powder**
1 **teaspoon baking soda**
1 **tablespoon finely ground dried lavender leaves**
1 **teaspoon dried lavender bud powder (optional)**

Mix together all ingredients. Store in an airtight container.

To use: Pour or spoon a small amount of the powder into your palm, and add a little water to form a paste. Massage into your scalp and throughout your hair. Rinse well and follow with a good conditioner.

Lavender Rice Flour Dry Shampoo

Dry shampoos are popular during times when you need to quickly clean your scalp and you do not have access to water or do not want to take a full shower. They are perfect for travel and after workouts. Dry shampoos also work to remove odors from your hair and freshen the scalp. If you have darker hair, you may want to use cacao powder in place of the rice flour, or a combination so that any leftover shampoo is not visible. It also gives a nice scent to the product. **Yield: 5 ounces**

> ½ cup rice flour or cacao powder
> 1 teaspoon baking soda
> 1 tablespoon borax powder
> 1 teaspoon dried lavender buds

In a food processor or blender, mix together all ingredients until you have a fine powder. Pour into a clean, dry container.

To use: Make sure you are either outside, over a sink, or standing on a towel, as this can be a bit of a messy first-time process.
Massage the powder directly into your scalp and through the hair.
Leave the powder on for 10 to 15 minutes to absorb impurities.
Vigorously brush your hair.

Lavender Vinegar Hair Rinse

Lavender vinegar diluted in water makes a cleansing hair rinse that will improve the condition of your scalp and encourage healthy hair. This antibacterial rinse will also soothe your scalp. **Yield: 8 ounces**

> 1 tablespoon dried lavender, or
>   2 tablespoons fresh lavender buds
> 1 cup apple cider vinegar
> 1 cup purified water

In a clean jar or bowl, add the lavender, and pour the vinegar and water over it. Let sit for several hours or overnight. The vinegar will turn a lovely pink shade. Strain and pour into a clean container.

To use: Add 1 tablespoon lavender vinegar to 1 cup water. After shampooing your hair, pour this rinse over and massage into your scalp. Rinse well with warm water.

Note: Never use straight vinegar on your hair or skin.

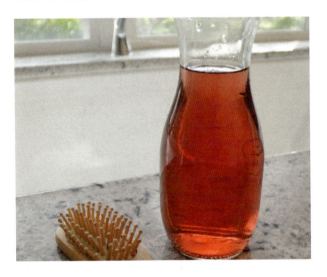

Lavender Mouth Rinse

Lavender leaves freshen the breath and clean and disinfect the gums. This is a mild, almost tasteless mouth rinse that has an airy floral fragrance. You can also use this as a skin freshener or after-bath

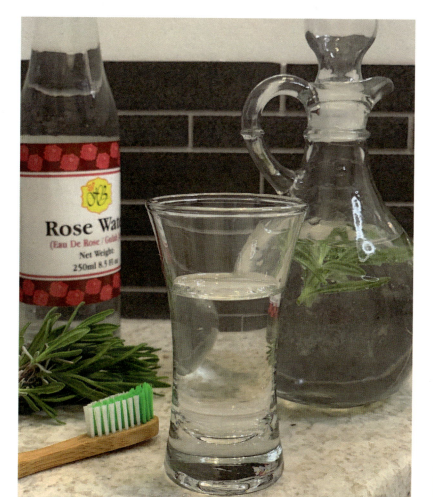

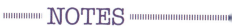

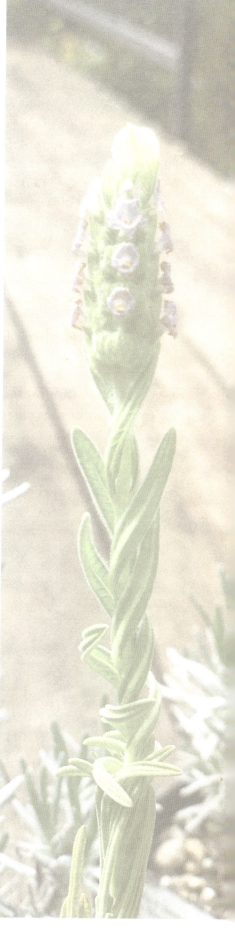

splash. This is especially helpful when you are traveling and want to avoid carrying several different products. Both lavender and rosewater are naturally antiseptic.
Yield: 8 ounces

    1 tablespoon lavender leaves, fresh or dried
    1 cup boiling water
    2 tablespoons rosewater

Place the lavender leaves in a glass or ceramic dish, and pour the boiling water over them. Let this mixture steep for several hours, then strain and discard the leaves. Add the rosewater to the scented liquid. Stir well, and pour into a clean bottle.

To use: Pour a small amount into a clean glass, and rinse your mouth after brushing your teeth and gums.

Lavender Facial Scrub

This gentle facial scrub will freshen and stimulate your skin. I use it in the evening before going to bed. It can be used alone, or mixed with a bit of your favorite soap or facial cleanser. Sugar is gentle enough to use on delicate

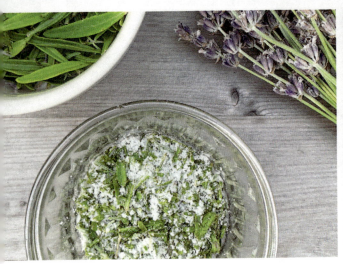
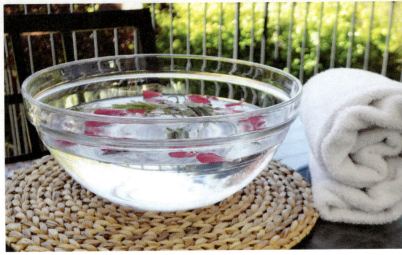

skin types. It is not as abrasive as it may feel at first, since it slowly dissolves as you wash with it. Use a combination of dried lavender buds and leaves, if you would like. Experiment by adding other dried herbs such as basil, rose, or chamomile to your mixture. **Yield: 8 ounces**

¼ **cup dried lavender buds and leaves**
1 **cup granulated or fine-grain raw sugar**

In a clean, dry glass jar, alternate layers of the sugar and dried lavender. Cover with a tight-fitting lid or beeswax wrap, and place in a dry spot for a few weeks.
When the sugar is scented to your liking, simply shake or stir the jar gently to mix. If you prefer, strain out the dried lavender bits using a fine mesh or piece of screen. Store in a clean, dry container.

To use: Pour a small amount of the scrub into the palm of your hand, and mix with water or your favorite cleanser. Massage into damp skin in a circular motion, then rinse well with warm water.

Lavender Rose Facial Steam

A facial steam is a good way to deep cleanse your pores. The heat and humidity gently open the pores, cleansing the skin of impurities. Fresh herbs and flowers, such as lavender and rose, help soften and clean your skin.

Please note: Steaming is not recommended for badly blemished or troubled skin. It can aggravate the condition by stimulating blood vessels and activating oil glands. If you have a continuing skin problem, check with a physician before trying. **Yield: 16 ounces (1 facial steam treatment)**

2 **cups water**
¼ **cup fresh lavender flowers and leaves**
¼ **cup fresh rose petals**

In a covered, medium-sized saucepan, bring water to a boil. Remove from heat, add the flower petals, and stir. Let the mixture sit for 5 minutes. Pour the hot floral water into a large bowl. Lean over the bowl, at least 12 inches from the surface, and drape a towel over your head to form a tent. Close your eyes and let the steam rise over your face for 5 minutes. Rinse with cool water and pat dry.

Note: Experiment with other flower petals and herbs, such as camellia, elderflower, basil, and rosemary.

Lavender Hand Cream

After a day spent in the garden, this rich cream is a welcome treat for your hardworking hands. I also like to massage it into my hands before gardening,

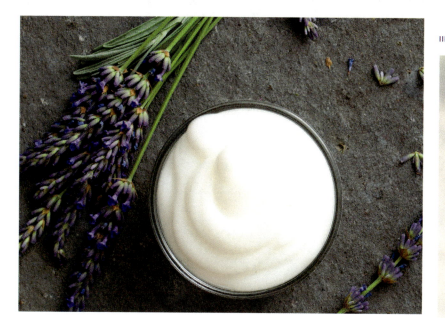

and then put on my garden gloves for an extra layer of protection. The dark sesame oil has only mild UV-protective properties, and should not be used in place of a good quality natural sunscreen. The scent of lavender is also a natural insect repellent. **Yield: 4 ounces**

> 3 tablespoons grated beeswax or emulsifying wax
> ½ cup dark sesame oil
> 1 tablespoon coconut oil
> 1 teaspoon honey
> 2 tablespoons strong lavender tea
> 2 to 3 drops lavender essential oil
> ⅛ teaspoon baking soda

Combine all ingredients in a heat-resistant glass container or double boiler. Heat gently on the stovetop, without boiling, over a water bath until all the wax and oils are melted, stirring well. Pour the melted mixture into a container or jar, and allow it to cool completely. Stir again when the mixture has cooled for a thick, rich cream.

To use: Massage a small amount into clean skin.

Lavender Foot Bath

Not everyone takes baths, or even has a bathtub in their home, but anyone can take foot baths. Foot baths are perfect for comforting and treating your whole body. They also help soothe your feet and remove rough skin spots. Abraham Lincoln was famous for saying, "If my feet don't feel good, I don't feel good," and this is so true. Lavender and thyme, as naturally antiseptic and comforting herbs, make a good combination in

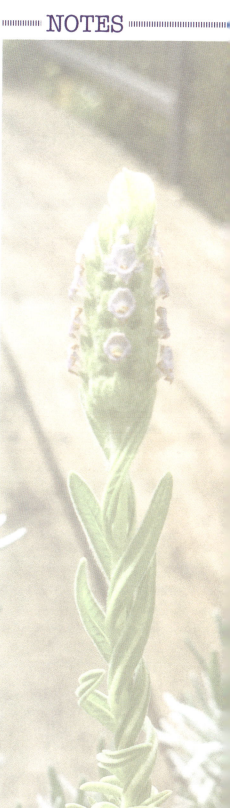

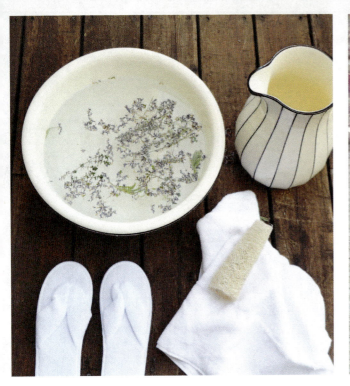
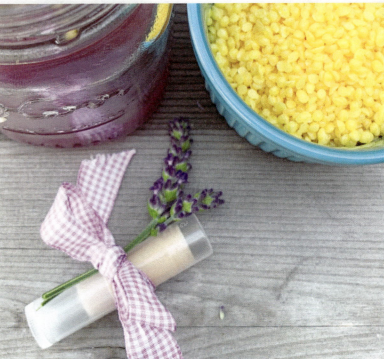

this recipe. After soaking for at least 10 minutes, use a natural pumice stone or luffa sponge to smooth your feet and remove rough skin. **Yield: 64 ounces (enough for one foot bath)**

> **2 quarts warm water**
> **¼ cup baking soda**
> **¼ cup Lavender Vinegar (see Page 43) or white vinegar**
> **1 tablespoon fresh lavender flowers and leaves**
> **1 tablespoon fresh thyme leaves**

Fill a tub or large plastic pan with warm water. Stir in the baking soda, vinegar, and fresh herbs. The water will fizz and bubble when the soda and vinegar are combined.

To use: Soak your feet for 15 to 20 minutes. Pat dry and massage them with a rich natural oil or cream.

Lavender Lip Balm

This is one of my favorite beauty recipes because it can be used for just about everything. Of course it works perfectly for protecting and soothing your lips, but it also works as a mini lotion bar, and can be used to treat dry cracked cuticles on your hands, insect bites, and minor cuts and scrapes. Simply rubbing a small amount on your temples can also calm a headache. I have a friend who applies it in the evening to help her get a better night's sleep. This recipe makes a large batch. If you only want a few tubes, simply change the amounts from cups to teaspoons. To experiment with natural colors, try a pinch of powdered purple sweet potato or red beetroot powder. **Yield: 8 ounces (30 to 40 tubes)**

> **½ cup lavender-infused coconut oil**
> **½ cup grated natural beeswax**
> **1 teaspoon apricot kernel oil**
> **1 to 2 drops lavender essential oil (optional)**
> **Powdered purple sweet potato (also called "ube"), or powdered red beetroot (optional)**

In a double boiler, combine all ingredients. Using medium heat, warm mixture gently over a water bath. Stir until the oil and beeswax are completely melted and well-mixed. Pour into lip balm tubes or tins and let cool until solid.

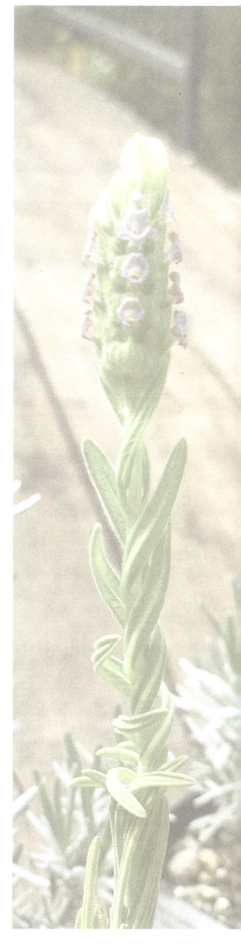

To use: Spread on your lips, or apply to minor burns, bites, and cuts.

Feel Better Lavender Bath Tea

When I feel a cold coming on, I immediately gather up my favorite cold-fighting herbs, such as lavender, rosemary, ginger, and eucalyptus, to make this fragrant bath blend. Simply fill a muslin bag or cotton square with the dried herbs and toss in your tub. After soaking in the fragrant water (until the water turns cool), wrap yourself up in a warm blanket with a strong cup of lavender tea. **Yield: 3½ ounces**

> 2 tablespoons dried lavender buds and leaves
> 2 tablespoons dried rosemary leaves
> 1 tablespoon chopped fresh ginger root,
>   or ½ tablespoon dried ginger
> 2 tablespoon dried eucalyptus leaves,
>   or 4 to 5 drops eucalyptus essential oil

Mix together all ingredients and place inside a large muslin tea bag or square of cotton fabric. Secure your bundle by tying up the ends with string.

To use: Toss the bundle into the warm water while filling the tub. Squeeze the bundle and place it behind your neck as you relax in the tub.

Note: Alternatively, add the herbs directly to the bath water. However, after the bath, the used herbal leaves and flowers remain. I don't recommend this method if you are too ill to clean the bathtub.

Relaxing Lavender Oatmeal Soak

Perfect for relaxing and soothing dry, sensitive skin, this soak contains oatmeal, baking soda, and lavender, all of which have healing properties. All skin types can use this recipe. The soak is especially soothing for those suffering from a bad rash, sunburn, or insect bites. Put the bath powder inside a piece of natural cotton or a muslin tea bag for easier cleanup. **Yield: 28 ounces**

> 1 cup dried lavender buds
> 2 cups whole oats
> ½ cup baking soda

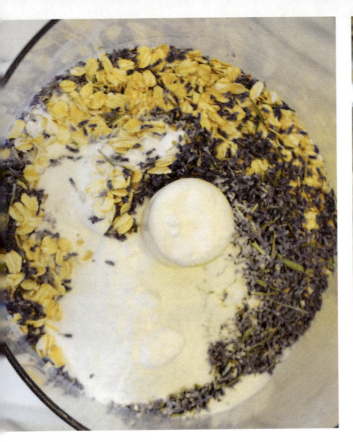

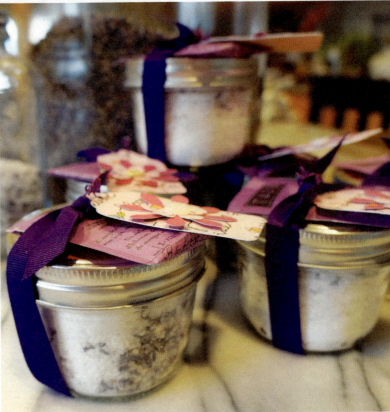

Place all the ingredients inside a food processor or blender; grind into a smooth, fine powder with the consistency of whole-grain flour. Pour the powder into a clean, airtight container.

To use: Pour in ½ cup as you fill the tub.

Note: Alternatively, fill a muslin tea bag or tie up the mixture in a square of cotton fabric, and toss it in the tub.

Lavender Bath Salts

Bath salts are one of my easiest and most popular DIY recipes. They are fun to create, anyone can enjoy them, and they make welcome gifts. If you are not a bath lover, or don't own a bathtub, use them in a foot soak. Epsom salts are a rich source of magnesium, an essential component of healthy bodies and muscles. Sea salt will boost your circulation, and baking soda is well-known for detoxifying the body. I make these salts with just dried lavender and sometimes a drop or two of essential oil. Feel free to experiment with your favorite herbs and herbal combinations. **Yield: 16 ounces**

1 cup Epsom salts (magnesium sulfate)
½ cup sea salt or kosher salt
½ cup baking soda
2 tablespoons dried lavender buds and leaves
4 to 5 drops lavender essential oil

In a large glass or ceramic bowl, mix together all the ingredients. Stir well and spoon into a clean container or muslin bag.

To use: Add ½ to 1 cup salts to your bath as you fill the tub. Soak for 15 to 20 minutes.

Lavender Bath Bombs

My grandmother's "bath fizzies" were similar to these. When I visited, I loved how they fizzed and exploded in the bath.

Nowadays these are called "bath bombs," and they're a bit larger than those I remember. The principle is the same; they deliver soothing salts and fragrant oils in an entertaining way.

When the bombs are dropped into a tub of water, the baking soda and citric acid combine, creating a chemical reaction that releases fizzy carbon dioxide bubbles.

Epsom Salts

Epsom salts, also known as magnesium sulfate, were first discovered in Epsom, England. When dissolved in water, the essential element, magnesium, is absorbed through your skin to increase circulation, warm tired muscles, and help you relax and sleep better at night. Used as a foot bath, Epsom salts help soften rough feet and soothe your whole body. Find Epsom salts in the first-aid aisle of any drugstore or grocery store.

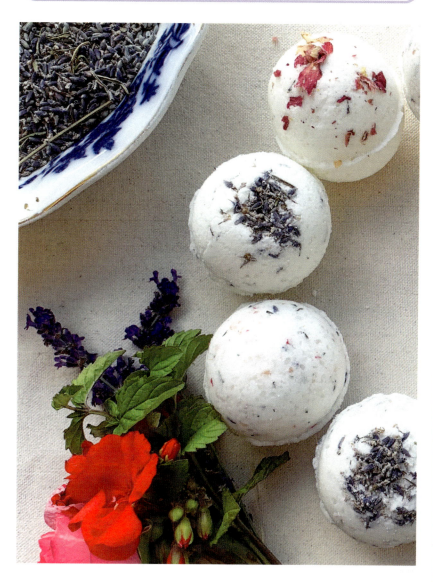

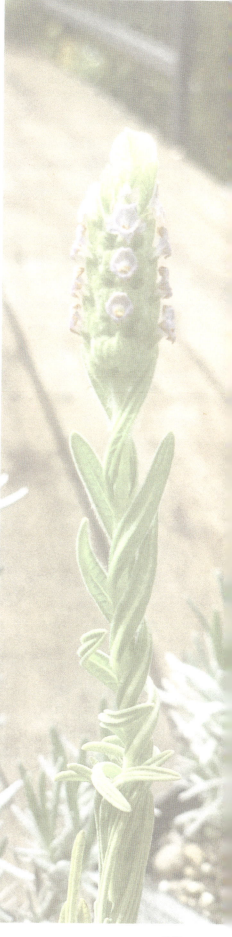

Yield: 16 ounces (about 6 bombs)

1 cup baking soda
1 cup citric acid powder
½ cup cornstarch
Powdered purple sweet potato (ube) for color (optional)
¼ cup coconut oil
3 to 4 drops lavender essential oil (optional)
1 to 2 tablespoons dried lavender buds

Bath Bomb Molds

Find bath bomb molds online, or at your local craft store. Search your home for possible molds; I use muffin tins, candy molds, bottoms of plastic drink containers, PVC pipe caps, paper cups, and gelatin tins. Use a bit of natural oil to grease the molds to make it easier to remove the finished product. Be creative! I once found an old children's sand toy shaped like a fish at the beach and still use that as a bath bomb mold.

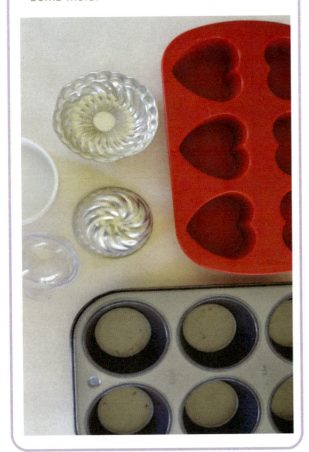

In a large bowl, combine the baking soda, citric acid, and cornstarch. For color, add the powdered sweet potato now. Also add some of the lavender buds if desired.

Melt the coconut oil in the microwave or stovetop over a water bath. Add a drop or two of essential oil, if desired.

Slowly add the oil to the dry mixture, stirring until you have a mixture that looks like wet sand. Sprinkle a bit of dried lavender into the bottom of your mold and then spoon in the bath bomb mixture, packing it tightly with the back of the spoon or with your fingers.

Let the mixture sit in the mold for 1 to 2 hours, or overnight.

Remove bath bombs from the mold and place them on a clean, dry surface; a cotton dish towel or a cookie sheet work well. Let the bombs sit for another day until nice and dry. Pack them inside a box or large jar.

To use: Drop one or two bath bombs into a tub of warm water and enjoy.

Eye Rest Pillow

To help cure dark circles under the eyes and brighten dull skin, a good night's sleep is essential. Sleep is also needed for good health; so why do so many of us miss out on snooze time?

An eye rest pillow is perfect for soothing tired eyes at night or during daytime naps. The natural flaxseeds give the pillow just the right amount of weight and help it conform to the shape of your face, blocking out light and giving you a feeling of peace and calm. Adding dried lavender gives your pillow a relaxing scent. Place the pillow inside a reusable bag in the freezer or refrigerator for a refreshing eye mask.

Yield: 1 eye rest pillow

Lavender Heating Pads

To create these pads, stitch up larger pillow shapes and fill them with lavender, along with flaxseeds, barley, or small-grain rice. Heat the pillow in the microwave for a minute or two, then place it on sore muscles. Use them as cold packs by placing them in the freezer. Use recycled fabric scraps or old clothes, and use natural fabrics. Some synthetics can melt when microwaved.

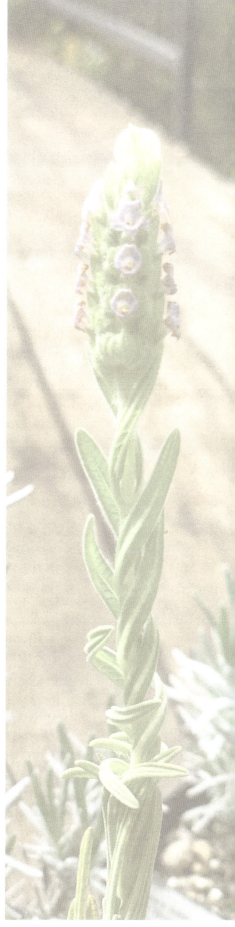

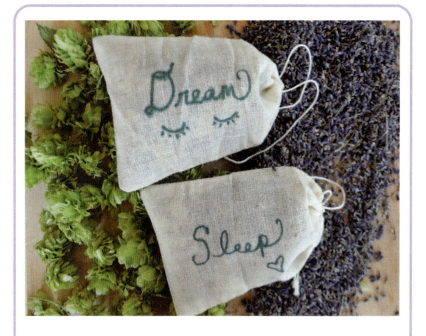

Lavender Dream Pillows

Centuries ago, many believed you could protect yourself from bad dreams by placing a combination of herbs in a bowl near your bed or stitched inside a small "dream pillow" placed under your pillow. Today, lavender still helps your mind and body relax. Use a couple tablespoons lavender and other herbs, and place inside a muslin tea bag, or stitch your own drawstring bag using the pattern on Page 104. They make nice gifts and are an easy project for a small group. Try these herbs in combination with lavender or on their own.

Hops: Relaxes and encourages sleep

Chamomile: Relaxes, good for children

Lemon Balm: Relieves stress, calms, relieves headaches

Rose: Relieves stress

Rosemary: Clears the mind, boosts memory

Marjoram: Improves sleep, relaxes the mind

Mugwort: Calms the mind, encourages good dreams

Peppermint: Refreshes, uplifts, and boosts mood

Lemon Verbena: Calms the nerves

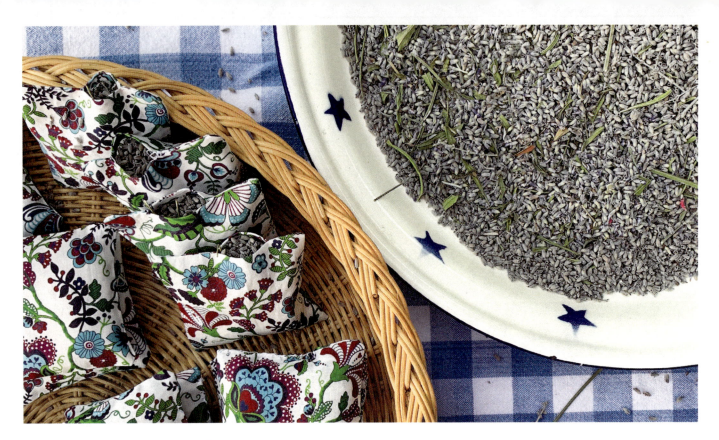

Flaxseeds
Natural fabric such as linen,
 cotton, or silk
1 to 2 tablespoons dried lavender
 buds

Cut out two pieces of fabric in either a rectangle or eye mask shape (see pattern on Page 105).

With right sides together, stitch around the shape, leaving a 1- to 2-inch opening. Turn inside out.

Add enough flaxseed to loosely fill the pillow. Add the lavender and shake gently to mix.

Stitch up the open end.

To use: Shake the pillow gently to release the lavender scent. Place over your eyes or behind your neck. Close your eyes and relax, focusing on the fragrance.

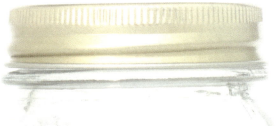

Upcycled Supplies

Shopping at yard sales and thrift stores will save you money, and they are great places to find reusable items. I look through my own kitchen cupboards, as well, for older pans, tins, and other kitchen equipment. The items may be past their prime for cooking, making them perfect for creating body-care products. Old cheese graters work on beeswax. Use saucepans, metal pitchers, and Pyrex measuring cups to create warm water baths to melt soap bases, waxes, and oils. Use old clothes and table linens made of natural fabrics to create lavender sachets, warming pads, and bath bags. And canning jar collections are great for storing products.

Beauty Recipe Notes, Inspiration, and New Ideas

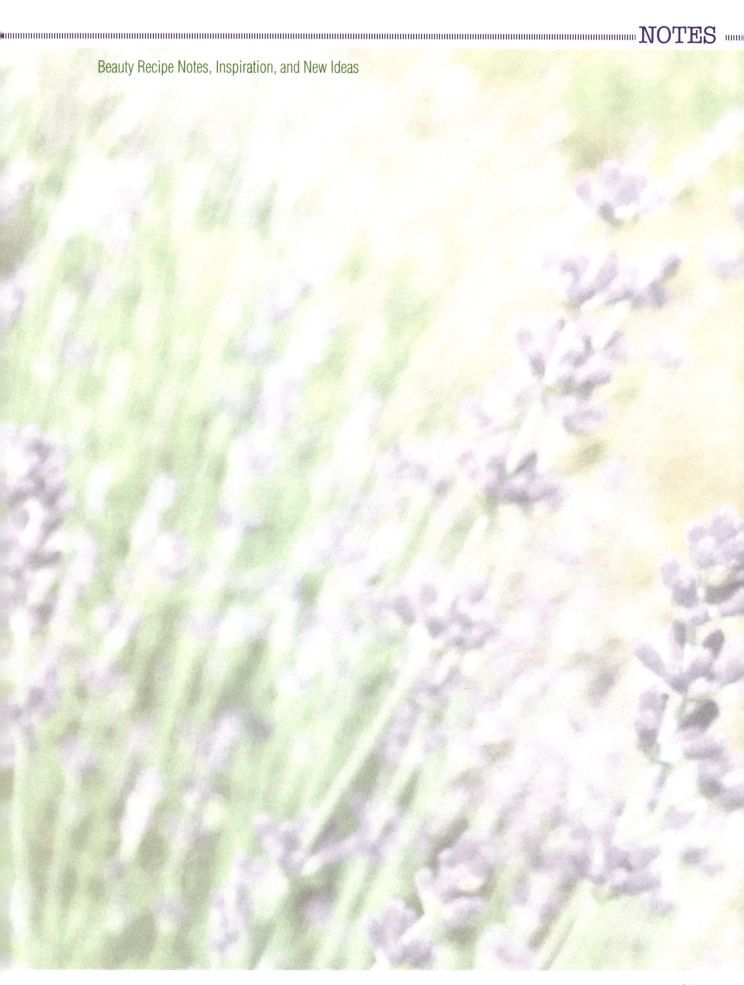

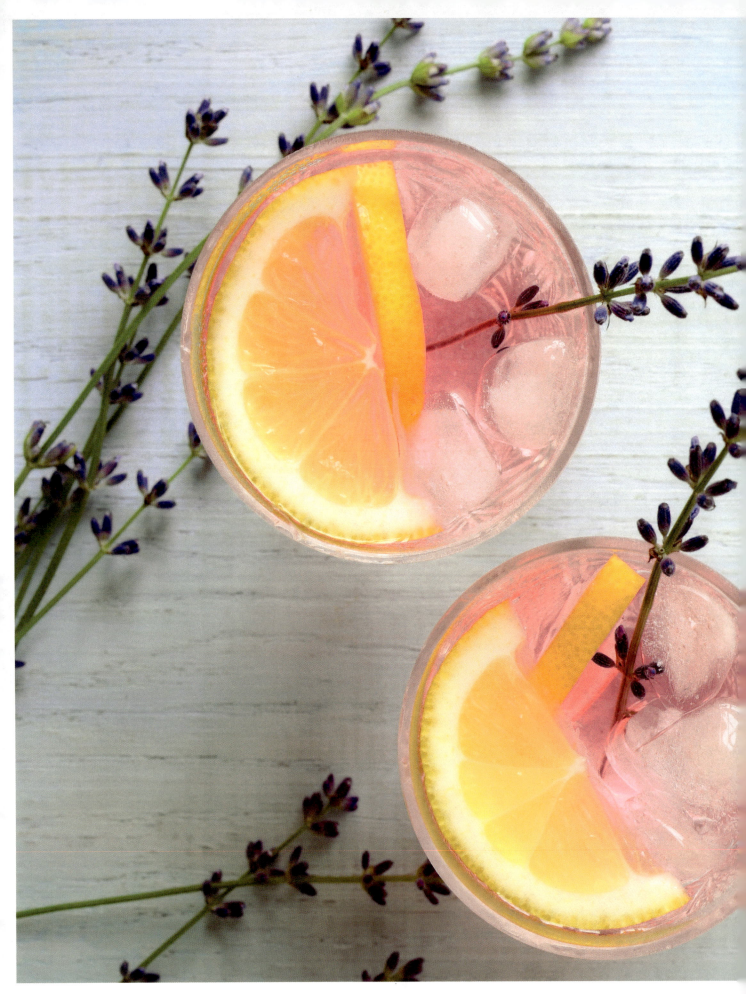

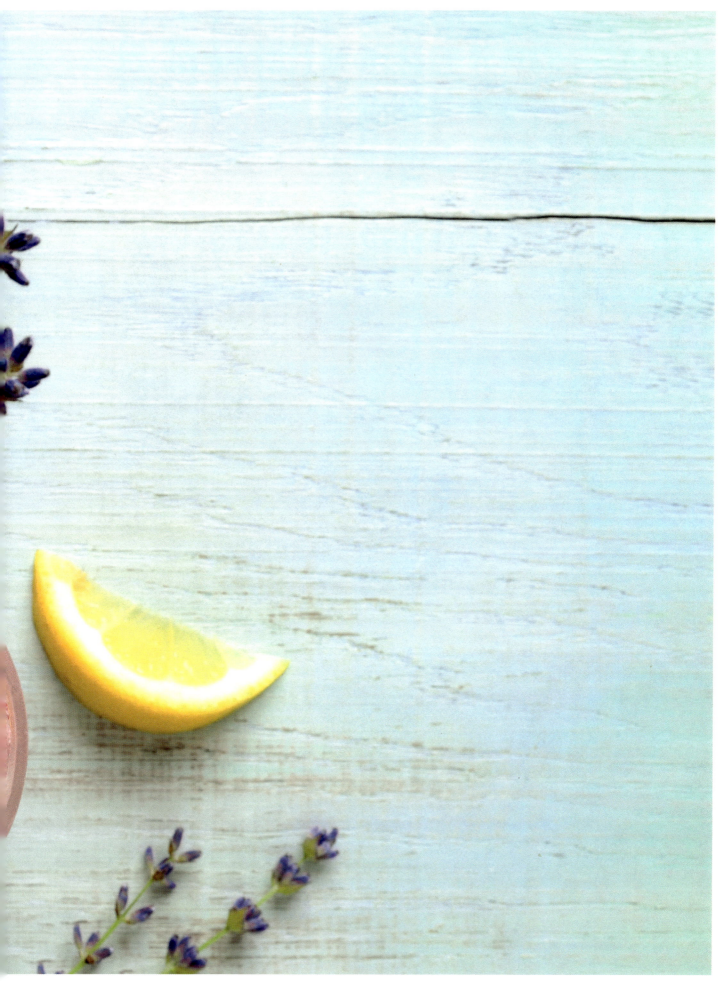

Chapter 3: Cooking With Lavender

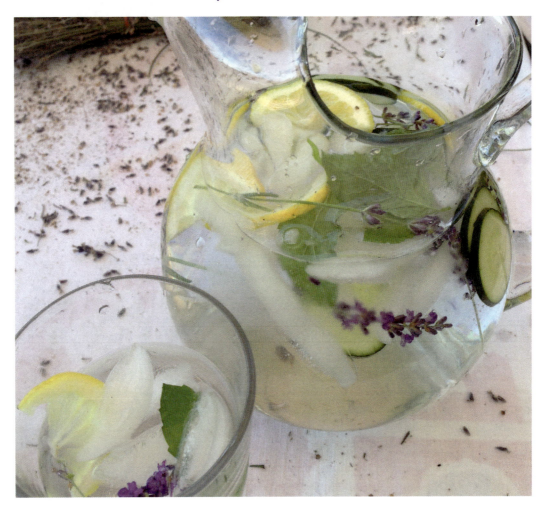

In addition to its strong floral scent, lavender's pretty purple buds and green leaves can be incorporated into your food. The essential oils within the buds add flavors of pine and rosemary, with a hint of citrus. From shortbreads to smoked meats, lavender will enhance a wide variety of recipes. Start by blending lavender with some of your other favorite culinary herbs or condiments, such as soy sauce, honey, or mustard. It also adds flavor to soft cheeses and marinades, and it mixes well with other herbs. One of the most famous French savory herbal blends, herbes de Provence (see recipe on Page 80), includes lavender in the mix.

Lavender adds flavor without adding extra salt or fat. A lavender simple syrup using fresh buds from my garden is one of my favorites. Use the recipe on Page 75 to flavor fruit salads, lemonade, or cocktails. Lavender syrup is also available for purchase at most lavender farms and some natural food stores.

Lavender honey is often for sale, which is usually an infused flavor, unless the beekeeper has a hive in the middle of a lavender field with no other blooms for miles. Make your own lavender honey by infusing it with dried buds.

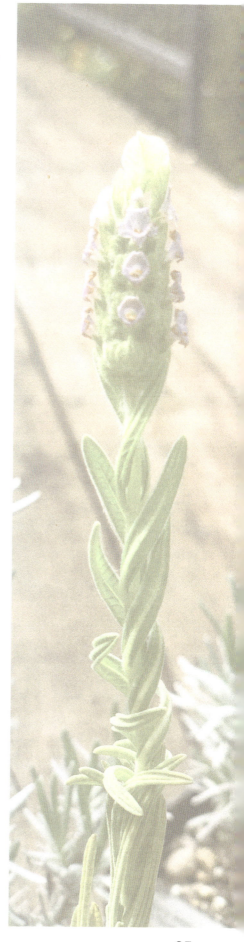

Sourcing and Harvesting Culinary Lavender

English lavender (*Lavandula angustifolia*) has the best flavor for cooking. French Lavender (*L. dentata*) and 'Provence' lavender (*L. dentata 'Provence'*) have the strongest flavors, and can sometimes overpower a dish. Spanish lavender (*L. stoechas*) is more astringent and has an almost a camphor-like flavor; I recommend avoiding this variety for flavoring foods. I also recommend cooks not use lavender essential oil. The method by which these oils are produced involves high heat and distillation, and they are not safe for ingestion.

When purchasing culinary lavender, look for dried buds and leaves with the culinary label. This tells you the flowers have been grown without any added sprays or fertilizers that could be transferred to your cooking. If you are growing lavender for culinary use or body-care products, mark your plants so you remember to not use any products on or around them that could be harmful to you and your family.

Lavender's essential oils are the most concentrated in the buds and flowers; for the strongest flavor, pick lavender stalks with buds just starting to open. When drying lavender for culinary use, choose a warm, dry, and dark spot with good airflow. Some people place paper sacks over their flowers, or place the flowers inside boxes to protect the buds from dust and small pests. I usually dry my flowers indoors, and once dry, I store the buds in a clean, amber or colored jar with a tight-fitting lid to preserve color and flavor.

Blooming Flavors

When you begin to cook with lavender, or add the herb to a favorite recipe, less is definitely more. It has a tendency to overwhelm a dish. Start with half the amount of dried lavender you think you'll need, and then increase it if you need to. Lavender flavors will also strengthen a recipe the longer the buds linger. This is known as the "lavender bloom."

The first time I made lavender shortbread cookies and sampled one of the first cookies from the batch, I could hardly taste the lavender; I thought the whole recipe was a flop. Then, by the time I was done baking them all, the cookies had cooled, and the lavender flavor was exquisite. So, remember to let your lavender sit or bloom to get the full flavor.

Lavender is especially wonderful in baked goods, which are often the first types of recipes people turn to when they begin adding lavender. Add it to cookies, muffins, quick breads, and cakes. If you are using it to make yeasted breads, just sprinkle it on top of your loaves for flavor since lavender's anti-bacterial properties can affect some yeasts, and subsequently, how your dough rises.

Culinary Infusions

Lavender also infuses well into natural oils, sugar, salt, alcohol, and honey. Simply add dried lavender to these ingredients, and let the mixture sit for a few days.

Lavender sugar is a versatile ingredient to keep on hand. To make lavender sugar, place a muslin tea bag filled with lavender buds inside a sugar jar and leave it for a few days. If you're happy with the flavor at this point, remove the tea bag. Some people just layer the sugar with lavender in a jar and this works well, too. With the second method, leave the lavender buds in the sugar until you're ready to use it, to ensure the flavor won't dissipate over time. Then, strain out the bits of lavender. For a quick and easy way to infuse your sugar, grind the buds with the sugar in a food processor or spice grinder.

Because of the high oil content of the buds, lavender infuses well into fats and oils. Try adding some fresh or dried buds to plain oils, butter, or other favorite condiments. When infusing oils to be stored, use dried lavender so no extra moisture is in your product.

When infusing lavender into alcohol and vinegar, the process begins almost instantly; you may only have to wait a few hours before you are satisfied with the flavor, at which point you can strain out the buds.

Lavender Sugar or Salt

Lavender Sugar is one of the easiest recipes to make, and it is a great multipurpose ingredient to have on hand. It adds a floral note to baking, and can be used on cinnamon toast, in coffee, or sprinkled on fresh fruit. I leave the buds inside the sugar jar until I am ready to use it, as a way to maintain the flavor. The same process works well with lavender-infused salt for making herbal seasoning blends.

Yield: 8 ounces

1 cup granulated sugar or kosher salt
1 tablespoon dried lavender buds

Experiment With Flavors

Any lavender can be used in the kitchen; English Lavender (*L. angustifolia*) works best. Experiment with different varieties; each one has a slightly different flavor or chemical profile. Some are floral and herbal, whereas others are citrusy, piney, even woodsy. Lavender pairs well with fruits, herbs, mild cheeses, nuts, sweets, and some meats. Lavender seems to complement smoked meats, and some people use the dried stems in their home barbecue grills or smokers to add flavor. If you are using lavender stems, make sure the stems are green or soak them first.

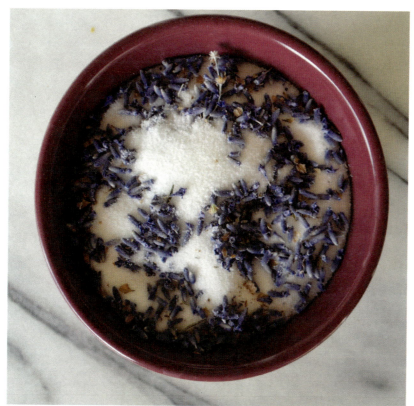

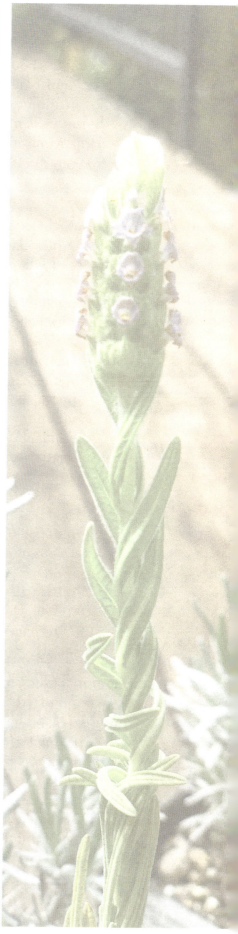

Place the sugar or salt in a large jar, and add the lavender buds. Cover with a tight-fitting lid and give the mixture a shake to distribute the lavender. Let sit for a few days.

If you are pleased with the scent and flavor, it is ready to use. If you wish for a stronger scent or flavor, let the mixture sit for a few more days, or add more lavender. Strain lavender buds out before using, unless you want lavender bits in your recipe.

Note: For gift-giving, leave the lavender buds in the sugar, and just write a note about straining before using.

Baking With Lavender

Lavender elevates a common box mix for brownies or cakes with its herbaceous flavor and floral notes. To add lavender, grind ½ teaspoon dried culinary buds in a clean spice or coffee grinder. Process until you have a smooth powder, and mix it into the brownie or cake mix. You can also find powdered lavender at some gourmet cooking shops and health food stores. Sprinkle the dried or fresh culinary buds onto frosted cupcakes, cakes, and cookies. Lavender blends well with other edible flowers, too, such as violets, rose petals, or geranium, and also with mint. Have fun experimenting with adding lavender to your favorite recipes.

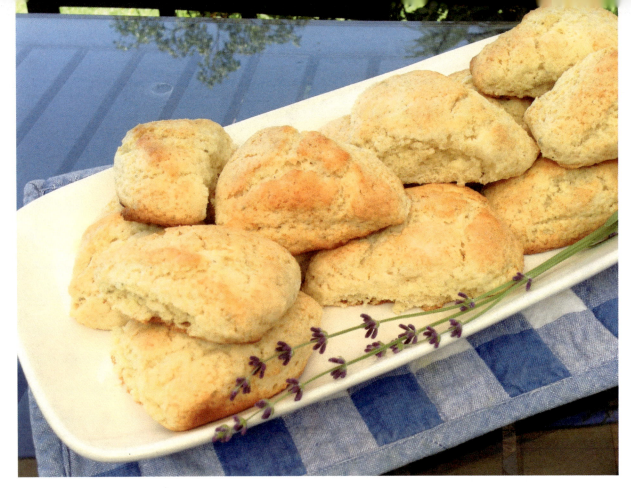

Lavender Scones

These sweet, fragrant scones pair wonderfully with a cup of tea. I usually prepare the dough, cut it into wedges, then bake what I need and freeze the rest for later. These scones make a quick and easy breakfast treat served with fresh fruit, homemade preserves, and some lavender tea or coffee. **Yield: 16 scones**

3 cups flour
¾ cup sugar
1 tablespoon baking powder
½ to 1 teaspoon dried lavender buds
1 teaspoon salt
½ teaspoon baking soda
¾ cup cold butter, cut into cubes
1 teaspoon vanilla
1 cup buttermilk

Preheat oven to 425 F. Line a large baking sheet with parchment paper; set aside.

In a food processor, place the flour, sugar, baking powder, lavender buds, salt, and baking soda, or mix the dry ingredients by hand in a large bowl.

Add the cold butter, and process or mix by hand until the mixture resembles coarse meal.

Add the vanilla to the buttermilk.

In a large bowl, add the wet ingredients to the dry ingredients, and stir until you have a rough dough. Transfer to a lightly floured surface and knead a few times, until a dough forms.

Divide the dough in half, and pat into two 8-inch rounds. Cut the rounds into 8 wedges each, and place the wedges on the prepared baking sheet. Brush with a little buttermilk, and bake for 13 to 15 minutes until golden-brown.

After removing from the oven, sprinkle with lavender sugar (see "Lavender Sugar or Salt" on Page 66), then place the scones on a wire rack to cool.

Note: Alternatively, add a bit of lavender to your favorite scone recipe. Lavender goes well with pumpkin, lemon, raspberry, and blueberry scones.

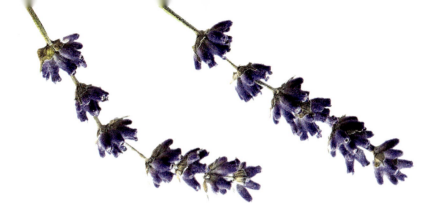

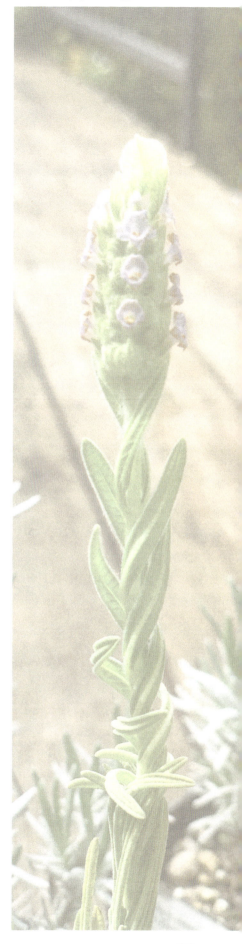

Lavender Shortbread Cookies

Lavender shortbread cookies are classic treats. I made this recipe for a lavender event we had in Kansas, and there were no leftovers! These cookies are easy to make with just a few ingredients, and they also keep well; they also freeze well. If you have a favorite shortbread recipe, add a small amount of lavender for a change. **Yield: about 2 dozen cookies, depending on size**

1 cup butter, softened
¼ cup granulated sugar
¼ cup powdered sugar
¼ teaspoon salt
1 cup all-purpose flour
1 cup cake flour
1 tablespoon fresh lavender, chopped, or
  ½ tablespoon dried lavender buds

In a stand mixer with a paddle attachment, cream together the butter, granulated sugar, powdered sugar, and salt until well mixed. You can also combine the ingredients by hand.

In a separate bowl, whisk together the two flours. Mix the flour mixture into the butter mixture. Add the lavender, and mix until just combined.

Place the dough onto a piece of parchment paper or plastic wrap, and form into a long roll, about 1 inch in diameter. Wrap up and refrigerate until firm (1 to 2 hours); I sometimes make the dough the day before I plan to bake the cookies.

To bake: Preheat the oven to 350 F. Line a cookie sheet with a piece of parchment paper; set aside.

Slice the dough into ¼-inch slices, place on the prepared cookie sheet, and bake until just golden-brown, about 12 to 15 minutes.

Remove from the oven, and let the cookies cool completely on a wire rack. Store in an airtight container or in the freezer.

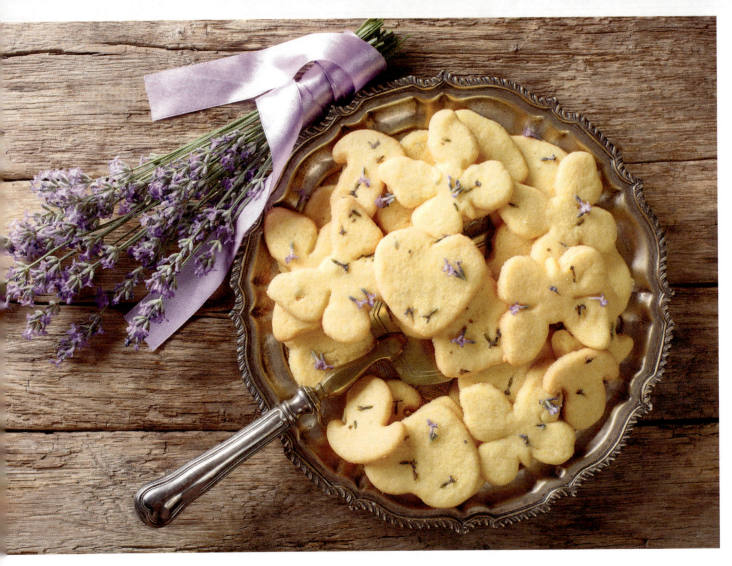

Lavender-Thyme Shortbread Cookies

This recipe is not as sweet as the Lavender Shortbread Cookies; however, the combination of lavender and thyme takes the flavor of these cookies up an herbal notch, and the olive oil lends them a healthful texture. They make a nice addition to an afternoon tea. Package them into gift boxes with some culinary lavender and a favorite tea blend. I sometimes make the dough a day ahead of time and store it in my refrigerator to bake the next day. Store the dough long-term in the freezer, where it will keep for up to a month. **Yield: approximately 6 dozen cookies**

   ½ **cup butter, softened**
   ¼ **cup olive oil**
   ½ **cup granulated sugar**

1 **tablespoon fresh thyme leaves, chopped**
1 **teaspoon salt**
1 **large egg, separated**
1¾ **cups flour**
2 **teaspoons culinary lavender buds, chopped**
1 to 2 **teaspoons baker's sugar**

Using a stand mixer or hand mixer, combine the butter, olive oil, and granulated sugar, and beat until smooth. Add the thyme, salt, and egg yolk. Save the egg white for brushing the tops of the cookies after baking.

Add the flour, and mix until you have a smooth dough.

Lay the dough out on a piece of plastic wrap or parchment and form into a long log. Wrap up and place in the refrigerator until firm, at least a hour.

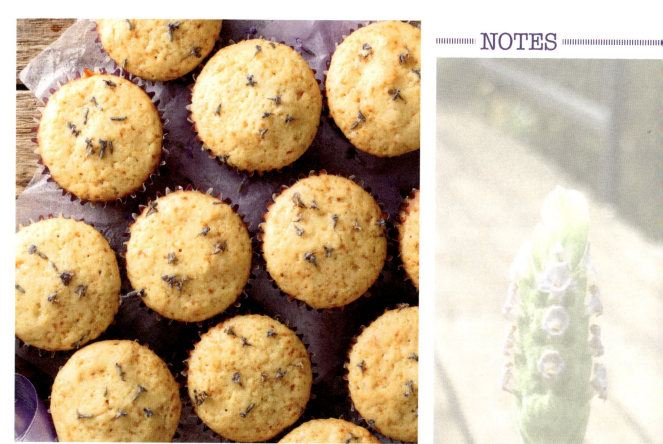

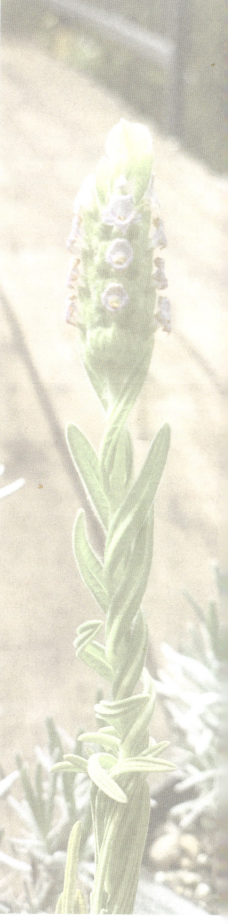

Preheat the oven to 350 F. Line a cookie sheet with parchment; set aside. Using a sharp knife, cut off ¼-inch slices of cookie dough, and lay them on the prepared cookie sheet. (Alternatively, roll out dough and use small cookie cutters for different shapes of cookies.)

Mix the lavender and baker's sugar. Lightly brush the tops of the cookies with egg white, and sprinkle with the lavender sugar mixture. Bake for 10 to 12 minutes until golden-brown. Do not overbake.

Place the cookies on a wire rack to cool.

Lemon Lavender Muffins

Lavender combines well with citrus, and some lavender varieties even exude a note of citrus flavor in their buds. Bake these muffins in mini-muffin tins and serve them when hosting a tea or as a sweet treat for a lavender brunch. Try using the citrus-lavender sugar blend in other recipes, or in your tea. Use it to glaze muffins, then sprinkle them with lavender buds and lemon zest for special treats. **Yield: 24 mini muffins, or 12 regular-sized muffins**

Lavender Citrus Sugar:
1 cup sugar
1 teaspoon dried lavender buds
1 teaspoon fresh lemon zest

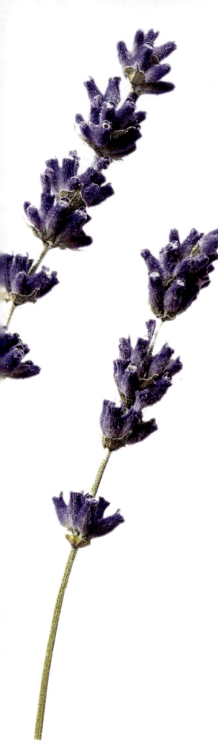

Muffins:

½ cup Lavender Sugar or Lavender Citrus Sugar
½ cup butter (one stick)
2 eggs
½ cup honey
½ cup almond milk or whole milk
2 tablespoons fresh lemon juice
1 teaspoon vanilla
1½ cups flour
½ teaspoon salt
1 teaspoon baking powder
¼ teaspoon baking soda

Lemon Glaze

1 cup powdered sugar
1 teaspoon fresh lemon juice
1 tablespoon almond milk or whole milk

For Lavender Citrus Sugar: In a food processor or blender, mix the sugar, lavender, and lemon zest until well-blended. This releases all the essential oils from the flower buds and citrus peel to flavor your sugar.

For Muffins: Preheat your oven to 350 F. Using an electric mixer, beat together the infused sugar, butter, and eggs until creamy. Beat in the honey, milk, lemon juice, and vanilla.

In a separate bowl, whisk together the flour, salt, baking powder, and baking soda. Add the dry ingredients to the butter mixture, and stir until just combined.

Spoon into greased muffin tins and bake until golden on top. For mini-muffins, bake about 10 to 12 minutes. For regular-sized muffins, bake 18 to 20 minutes.

Let cool completely, and sprinkle with more Lavender Sugar, or top with Lemon Glaze and flower buds.

For Lemon Glaze: Whisk together all ingredients until smooth.

Lavender Beauty Balls

I love to make these beauty balls, as I call them, because they contain two superfoods for beauty: cacao powder and walnuts. Magnesium-rich cacao beans provide the chocolate base. Walnuts are a good source of magnesium, as well as omega-3 fatty acids. I like to keep a supply in my freezer for a healthful sweet treat. This recipe contains only a tiny amount of lavender. If you wish for a stronger flavor, feel free to increase it, and also experiment with other herbs and spices, such as

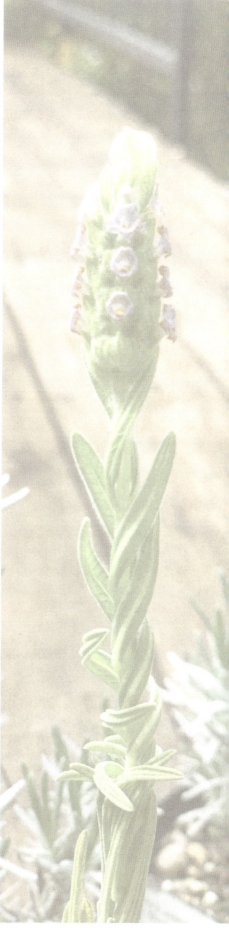
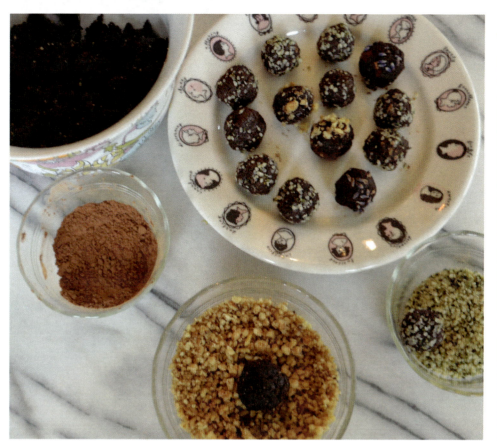

cinnamon and chamomile. Roll these balls in more finely chopped walnuts or cacao powder. **Yield: approximately 3 dozen beauty balls**

> 1 cup chopped pitted dates
> 1 cup chopped walnuts
> ¼ cup cacao powder
> ½ teaspoon vanilla
> ⅛ to ¼ teaspoon dried culinary lavender buds
> 2 tablespoons water
> 1 to 2 tablespoons finely chopped walnuts,
>   or cacao powder, for garnish

Place all ingredients, except garnish, in a food processor. Process until you have a thick mixture that holds together. You may need to add another 1 or 2 teaspoons of water. Place the mixture in a bowl, and leave in the refrigerator or freezer until firm (about 20 to 30 minutes).

Scoop out teaspoon-sized amounts, and roll into balls with your hands. Roll in nuts or cacao powder to coat. Place in an airtight container, and store in the freezer.

Lavender Sea-Salt Almonds

Our family traveled to Hawaii one year for a spring vacation and stayed on the island of Maui. My daughter, Lauren, and I went on an upcountry drive where we

Lavender Tea Blends

Create your own custom tea blends using favorite garden herbs and spices. When shopping for teas at the grocery store or in tea shops, read the labels of blends you enjoy. You may discover a new combination. I found one featuring lavender, chamomile, and cinnamon that I enjoy in the evenings. Here are a few other favorite blends to try:

Sweet Dreams: Lavender, Mint, Chamomile, and Rose
Energizing: Green Tea, Lavender, and Lemon Peel
Fruit Tea: Hibiscus Tea, Fresh Berries, and Lavender
Colorful: Butterfly Pea Tea, Lavender, and Chamomile This combination makes a blue tea. For a magical color change, add a bit of lemon, and it will turn a lovely shade of purple.
Note: All of these tea blends can be served hot, or cold over ice.

discovered a lavender farm that served lavender coffee and scones. While we were there in March when the lavender was not yet in bloom, it was still beautiful; everything was so green and the views were amazing. I encourage you to visit a lavender farm off-season for a different perspective on the plants without the usual crowds. This recipe reminds me of that day at the farm where we bought some of their candied nuts. They are great for parties, or a hostess gift.

Yield: 16 ounces

> 1 teaspoon finely ground dried lavender buds
> 2 tablespoons sugar
> 1 teaspoon salt
> 1 pound marcona or raw almonds
> 3 tablespoons macadamia nut oil or olive oil

Preheat the oven to 300 F. Line a cookie sheet with parchment paper; set aside.

In a small bowl, mix together the lavender, sugar, and salt.

In another bowl, toss the almonds with the oil.

Spread the nuts onto the prepared cookie sheet. Bake until golden-brown, about 15 minutes.

Remove from the oven, sprinkle with the lavender mixture, and stir to coat. If desired, transfer the mixture to a bowl to make mixing a bit easier. Let cool completely and store in an airtight container.

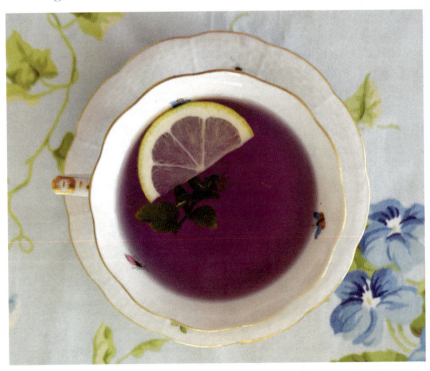

Lavender Tea

Lavender tea has been used for centuries to calm the body and mind, as well as to boost mood. Queen Victoria was known to have a cup of lavender tea every day. Lavender tea is simple to make from buds, with fresh or dried lavender flowers in the mix. Rich in vitamin C and vitamin A, lavender tea helps improve digestion after a meal or before bedtime. Most grocery stores carry lavender tea. Brew your own, by purchasing culinary lavender, or by using your own plants. **Yield: 8 ounces**

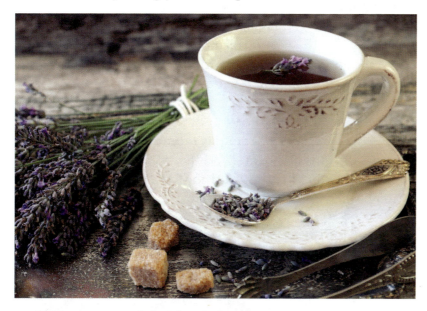

1½ **teaspoons dried lavender, or**
   1 **tablespoon fresh lavender buds**
8 **ounces boiling water**

Place the lavender inside a metal tea strainer or muslin tea bag, and place inside your teacup or teapot. Pour the boiling water over the plant buds and let steep for 10 minutes.

Strain or remove the lavender buds. Add lemon, cream, and sugar as desired.

Lavender Simple Syrup

Just as the name says, this recipe is simple. Add this classic ingredient to an endless number of drink and cocktail recipes, and experiment by infusing it with herbs and fruits. It's also a fitting garnish to fruit salads, oatmeal, yogurts, and pancakes. The basic recipe uses equal parts sugar and water heated until the sugar

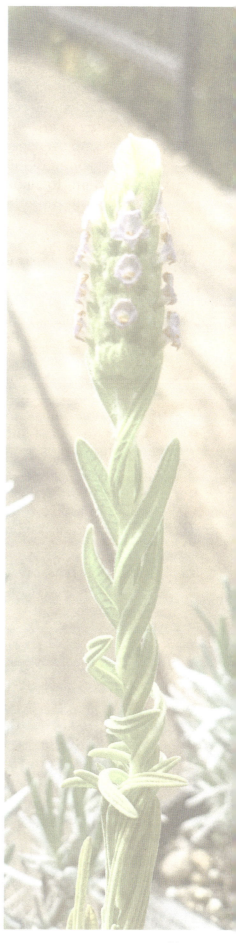

Host a Lavender Breakfast or Tea

Before any MOTHER EARTH NEWS Fair workshop, we host a lavender breakfast, which creates a relaxing start to a busy day. It gives people a chance to connect with local lavender farmers and garden groups. Because our kitchens are usually limited, we often serve everything outdoors. This is an easy menu that comes together quickly, and gives everyone a chance to sample a variety of lavender dishes. We sometimes have a "make and take" activity, such as starting plants, creating a bath salt, or filling a simple sachet. Use the invitation on Page 103 or create your own. Our menu includes:

Quiche with Herbes de Provence
Seasonal fruit salad with Lavender
  Simple Syrup
Tossed greens with lavender vinaigrette
Lavender Scones, Lemon Lavender
  Muffins, and quick breads
Lavender oatmeal with a variety
  of toppings
Lavender coffee, served with lavender
  cream and sugar
Lavender Tea (I often combine lavender
  and butterfly pea flowers)
Lavender Lemonade
Lavender Mimosas

Feel free to add your favorite dishes to this simple menu. I sometimes purchase quiches from a local shop, and whip up an easy sauce by mixing my herbes de Provence blend with sour cream. Depending on the time of year, we serve the tea iced with the option of mixing it with equal parts lemonade. For the mimosas, set up a bar with assorted fresh fruit juices, champagne, and lavender simple syrup. Lavender jams and honey also add a nice touch. We sometimes give out small jars or simple sachets of lavender.

dissolves, and then it's cooled and stored. For natural color, add a few fresh blackberries or blueberries. You can also purchase simple syrups at lavender farms and specialty food stores. **Yield: 16 ounces**

> 1 cup water
> 1 cup sugar
> 2 tablespoons culinary lavender
> 8 to 10 fresh blueberries or blackberries,
>   crushed

Place all the ingredients in a saucepan, and cook over medium heat. Stir constantly until the sugar is completely dissolved.

Remove from heat, and let cool completely to allow the lavender flavor to infuse into the syrup. Strain your syrup into a clean bottle with a tight-fitting lid.

Store in the refrigerator for 2 to 3 weeks.

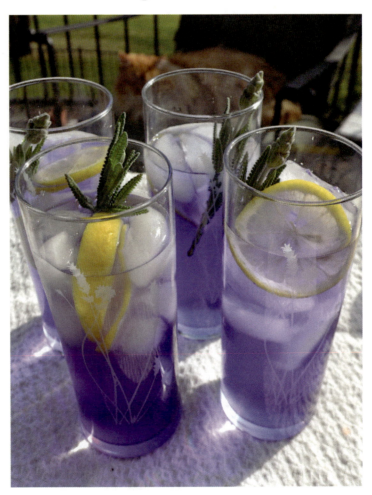

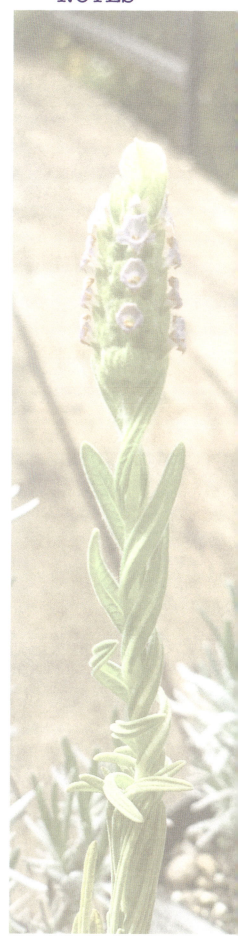

Lavender Lemonade

This has become a classic, popular drink served at lavender festivals and events across the county. The lavender combines well with fresh citrus. Though this recipe makes a basic lemonade, try replacing the water with herbal teas, such as chamomile or mint, or add butterfly pea to turn it purple! (See "Butterfly Pea Tea" recipe below.) You can also add fruit juices such as blueberry or pineapple, or spike your lemonade by turning it into a cocktail! **Yield: 1 quart (32 ounces)**

- **4 cups water or herbal tea**
- **1 cup sugar**
- **2 tablespoons dried lavender buds or**
  ¼ cup fresh lavender buds
- **1 cup fresh lemon juice**
- **1 fresh lemon, sliced, and a few sprigs of fresh lavender, for garnish**

Butterfly Pea Tea

The flowers of the butterfly pea vine (*Clitorea ternatea*) make a beautiful electric-blue tea. This magical Asian vine with bright-blue flowers is also known as Asian pigeonwings, bluebellvine, or Darwin pea. You may find the plant at your local nursery, or buy seeds online. In warmer climates, it's a perennial vine, and it's an annual in cooler climes. The dried flowers are usually sold in the tea section of most natural food stores.

Its flowers create a beautiful indigo-colored tea that's pH-sensitive; if you add an acid to it, such as vinegar or lemon juice, it instantly turns from blue to purple, or even pink. As a healthful hot or cold drink, this antioxidant-rich tea offers stress-relieving properties similar to chamomile tea. I love to add it to lemonade for a lovely shade of purple, and I also add it to scented play dough (see "Play Dough" recipe, Page 95) to create a lovely lavender-colored dough. You might see it featured in commercial anti-aging products as well. I like to use it in hair rinses, facial masks, and in skin toner recipes.

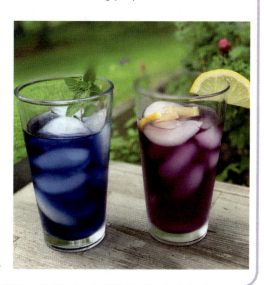

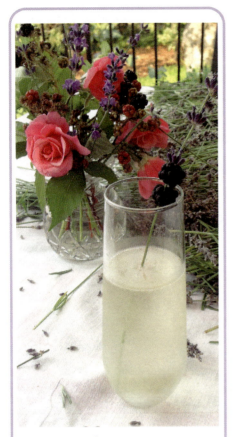

Lavender Mimosas

Creating a mimosa using lavender can take several different routes. The classic brunch drink involves fruit juice, champagne, and a splash of simple syrup. Lavender simple syrup will take any mimosa recipe to the next level, and give it a bit of sophistication. At a workshop in Oregon, I learned a trick from one of my lavender friends. She used blueberry juice in her mimosa to create a gorgeous purple color. Her recipe is so easy: Put a few tablespoons fresh berry juice in a champagne flute, add a splash of lavender simple syrup, and top it all off with champagne. Use other fruit juices, such as raspberry or peach as you wish. Cheers!

In a saucepan, combine the water, sugar, and lavender. Heat, stirring constantly, until the sugar is completely dissolved. Let the mixture cool completely, then strain out the buds.

Add the lemon juice and stir well.

To serve, add fresh lemon slices and lavender buds to your pitcher, or to individual glasses filled with ice, and add your lemonade. Garnish with a fresh sprig of lavender. Store in the refrigerator.

Note: If you are short on time and don't want to make your own fresh lemonade, simply mix frozen lemonade from concentrate with a strong lavender tea in place of the water called for on the can. Add a few fresh lemon slices, and your almost-homemade lemonade is ready to be served.

Casino Royale Lavender Martini

In the Bond film *Casino Royale*, James creates a "vesper martini." He orders it made with the French aperitif wine, Lillet; vodka; and a slice of lemon peel. I have adapted this recipe using lavender. The herb pairs extremely well with both vodka and gin, and I think the James Bond character, Vesper Lynd, may like this version even better! Lillet can be found at most liquor stores. For a stronger lavender flavor, infuse your vodka or gin for this recipe. The flavors develop rather quickly, so only leave the dried buds in the alcohol for a few hours, then strain. **Yield: 3 ounces**

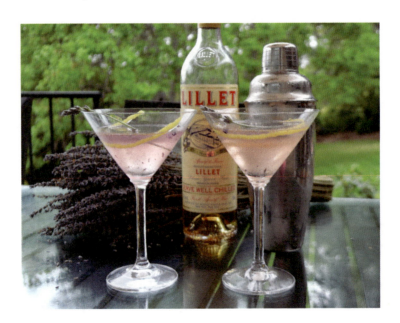

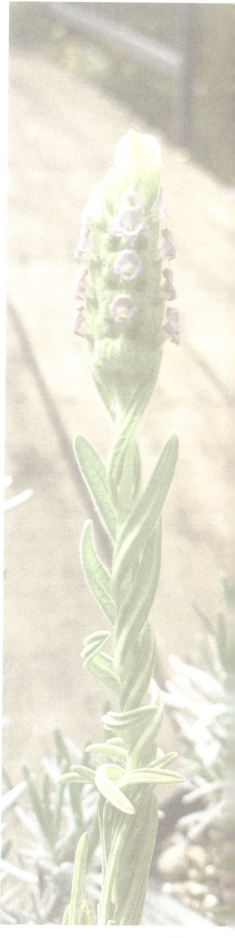
1 to 2 teaspoons fresh lavender buds
2 tablespoons lavender-infused vodka or gin
1 tablespoon Lillet blanc wine
Lemon peel
Fresh lavender sprig

In a cocktail shaker filled with ice, add the fresh buds, vodka, and wine. Shake well and strain into a cocktail glass. Remember the famous order: "Shaken not stirred."

Garnish with a large slice of lemon peel and a fresh sprig of lavender.

Note: Purchase lavender spirits from lavender farms and liquor stores if you'd rather not infuse your own.

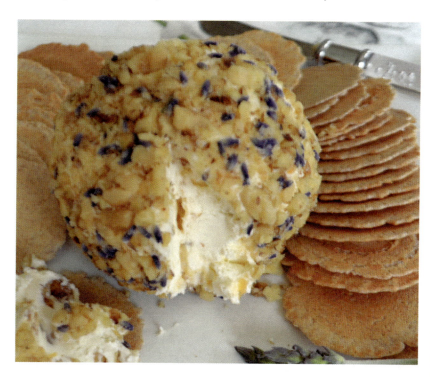

Lavender Cheese Ball

My mother always served a cheese ball with sliced fruits, crackers, and nuts at all of her holiday parties during my growing-up years. It was the classic appetizer of the 1950s, and my mother, a home economics major, knew the value of a good premade appetizer. It looks harder to make than it really is. This cheese ball is inspired by my childhood memory of my mother's recipe; it is easy to create, full of fruit and nuts, with a hint of lavender. It works well all on its own with some crackers, or as a welcome addition to a cheese board when entertaining.

Yield: 8 ounces

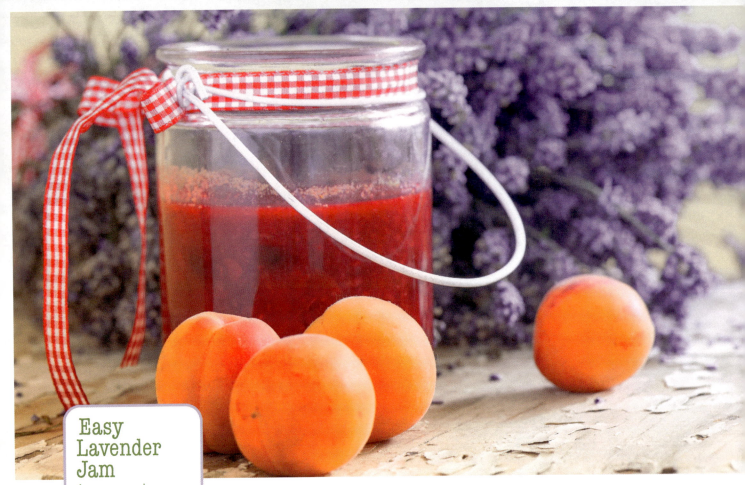

Easy Lavender Jam

An easy and quick recipe for creating a really yummy jam adds a delightful touch to toast and scones, when served with a cheese board, or as a topping for vanilla ice cream. Heat a cup of your favorite jam. I use peach or apricot, though any fruit jam or marmalade will work. Add 1 teaspoon dried lavender buds, and stir well. Heat the jam until it just starts to bubble; don't boil. Cover and let it sit for a few hours, the longer the better.

8 ounces cream cheese, softened
1 tablespoon lavender-infused apricot jam
1 tablespoon chopped dried apricots
½ cup + 1 tablespoon chopped walnuts or pecans, divided
1 teaspoon dried lavender

In a small bowl, mix together the cream cheese, jam, dried apricots, and 1 tablespoon nuts. Mix well, and spoon into a small bowl lined with parchment paper or plastic wrap. Place in the refrigerator until firm, about 30 minutes.

In a glass pie pan or dish, place the ½ cup chopped walnuts and sprinkle with the dried lavender.

Remove the cheese mixture from the refrigerator and shape into a ball. Roll the ball in the chopped nuts and lavender to coat. Return to the refrigerator for several hours.

Serve with sliced apples or crackers.

Herbes De Provence

This classic herbal blend originates from the Provence region of southeast France, well-known for its lavender fields. Several recipes can be found online, as well as herb blends for sale. Some variations use up to 11 ingredients. I like this recipe because it uses common herbs most of us can grow or purchase at a local market. It makes a nice seasoning alternative to

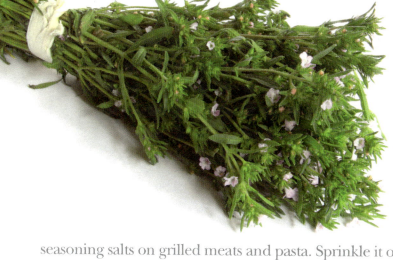

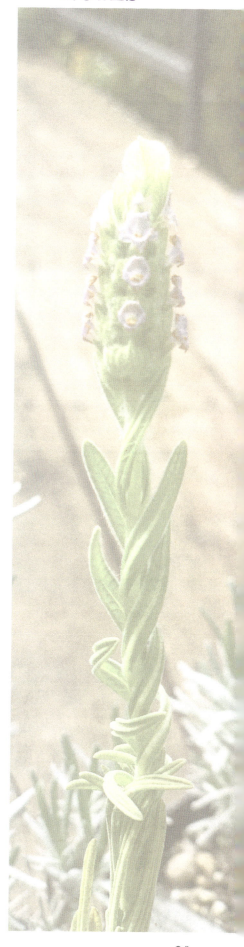

seasoning salts on grilled meats and pasta. Sprinkle it on deviled eggs, and mix it into sour cream and cream cheese. It also makes a nice gift from your garden. **Yield: 3 ounces**

> 2 teaspoons dried lavender buds
> 2 teaspoons dried thyme
> 2 teaspoons dried basil
> 2 teaspoons dried rosemary leaves
> ½ teaspoon dried summer savory
> ½ teaspoon dried marjoram leaves
> 2 teaspoons dried lemon peel or zest

Mix together all the ingredients by hand, or give them a quick whirl in the food processor or spice grinder. Store in a clean, dry, colored or amber jar with a tight-fitting lid to preserve color and flavor.

The Herb of Love

Summer savory *(Satureja hortensis)*, a peppery annual herb in the mint family, is also key ingredient in herbes de Provence blends. Sometimes called "the herb of love," ancient Romans believed this plant to be a natural aphrodisiac, and they used it in creating love potions. The plant has pale purple flowers that bloom in the summer. It makes a nice addition to a traditional herb or container garden.

Create Your Own Lavender Herb Blends

Lavender works well with a variety of herbs and spices. Create your own special blends to use when you cook. Use the chart on the next page to record the amounts used, and the variety of herbs that works well for you. Add your special blends to cream cheese, butter, oils, sauces, and cookies. Experiment with a small amount until you have a blend that appeals to you. Then you can go into production!

CREATE YOUR OWN LAVENDER HERB BLENDS

Name	Herbs Used and Variety	Other Ingredients	Amounts Used in Recipe	Yield Amount	Uses	Notes & Comments

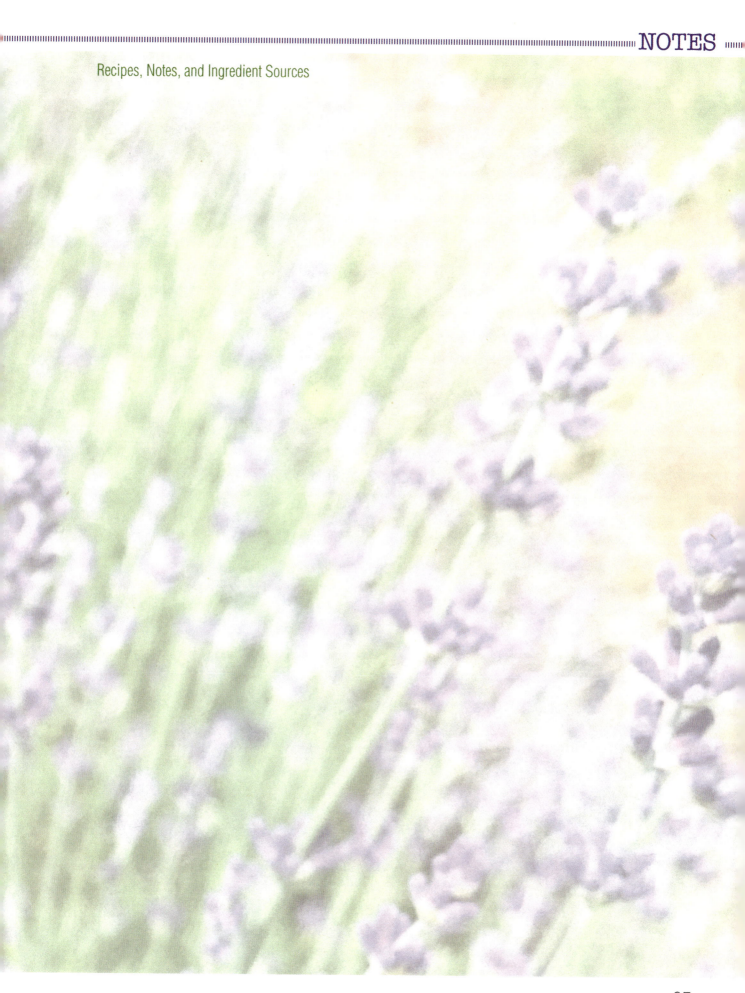

Recipes, Notes, and Ingredient Sources

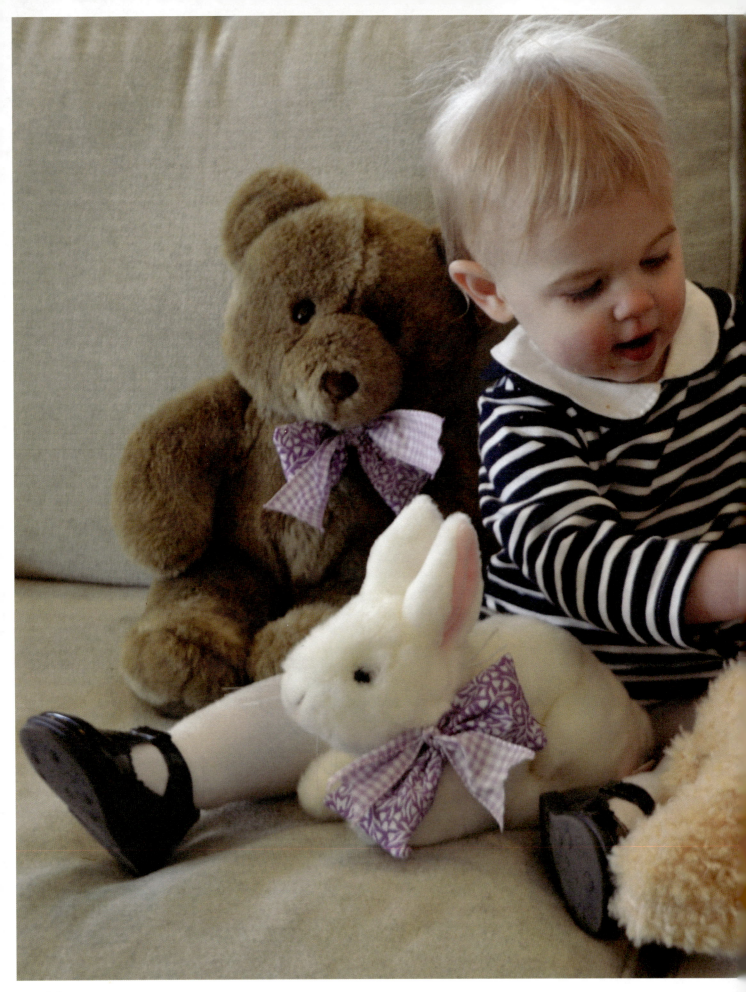

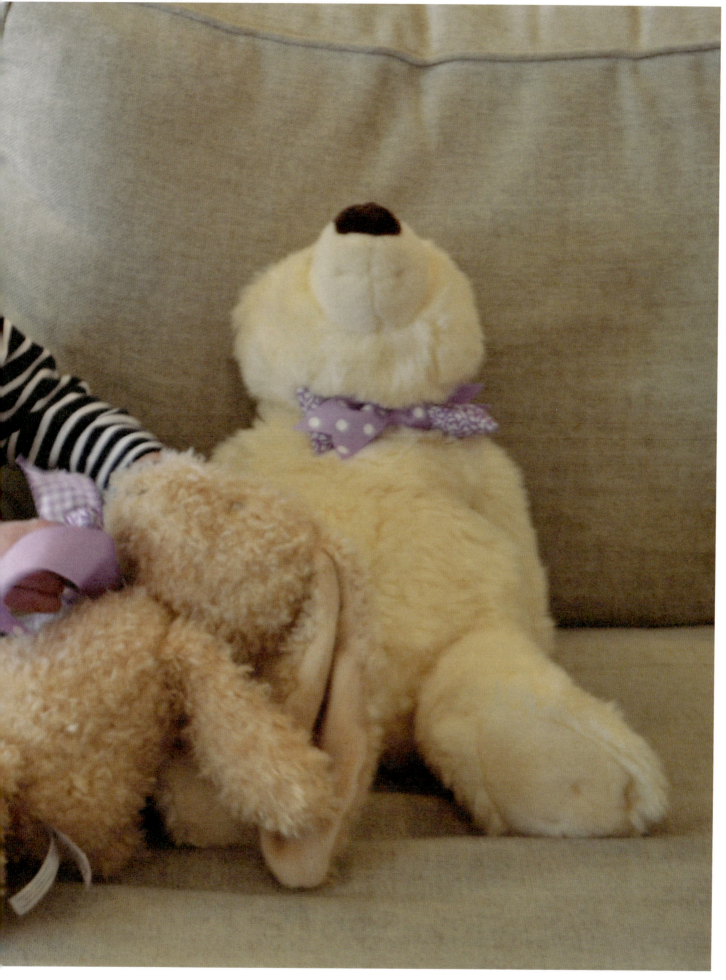

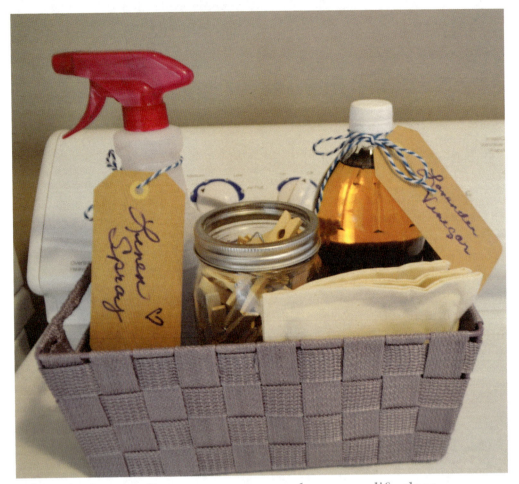

In this chapter, discover more ways to keep your life clean, comfortable, and creative with lavender. Using dried buds and common household ingredients, create your own lavender disinfectant sprays, scented sachets to keep fabric fresh in drawers and closets, and more. Also learn how to keep your pets healthy with this fragrant herb, which repels fleas and ticks, and keeps chickens clean, relaxed, and calm.

Get crafty with lavender by weaving it into wreaths, flower crowns, and wands. Discover the multiple ways to use and create sachets: as dream pillows, dryer fresheners, shoe inserts, and even as a calming toy for children. Use lavender oil to create your own scented products, such as candles and aromatherapy charms. Or, make your own oil by infusing it with lavender, or blending it with distilled oils.

All-Purpose Lavender Cleaner

Replacing toxic cleaning chemicals in your home with natural ingredients will not only save you money, it will also help improve your and your family's health and the environment. Here is basic cleaner recipe to get you started. Feel free to adapt the recipe to your own needs. **Yield: 16 ounces**

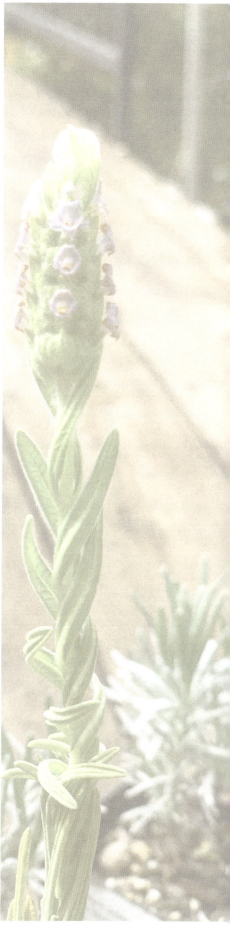

2 tablespoons white or Lavender Vinegar (Page 43)
1 teaspoon borax powder
Peel from 1 lemon
1 tablespoon dried lavender buds
2 tablespoons mild liquid soap, such as castile
2 cups water

Mix together the vinegar, borax, lemon peel, and lavender buds, and let sit for a few days to infuse. Strain the mixture, and pour into a clean container. Add liquid soap and water, and shake or stir gently to mix.

To use: Spray or wipe onto surfaces to clean and disinfect. Rinse with water.

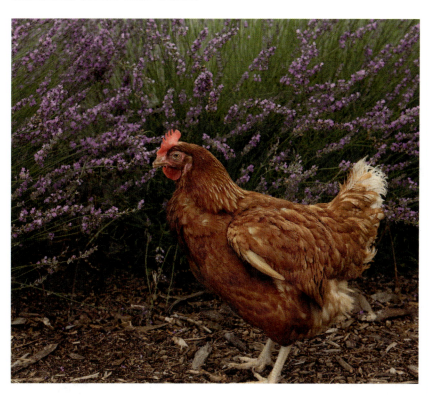

Chicken Coop Cleaner

You often see lavender growing near chicken coops; it helps repel bugs, and, when stems are added to nesting boxes, some believe it increases egg production by keeping the hens more relaxed. Chicken herbs sold in stores almost always include lavender.

This simple, all-natural cleaner helps deodorize and freshen your coop. It also works as an all-purpose cleaner for other household chores. Spot test some surfaces first, as vinegar is a mild acid. **Yield: 12 ounces**

Creating your own scented candles is a great way to repurpose old jars, teacups, used candle jars, and even glass bottles as homemade candle holders. My daughter, Marie, and I made dozens of "Lavender Wine Bottle Candles" to give as gifts one year. We collected used bottles from local restaurants, and purchased a bottle cutter to make the candle containers. When her friends used up the candles, they were delighted to reuse the containers again as small flower vases or planters! (Succulents do really well in recycled glassware.) If you don't want to purchase a bottle cutter, glass shops often will cut your bottles for just a small fee.

½ cup white vinegar
4 tablespoons dried lavender buds or ¼ cup fresh buds (leaves work, too)
1 to 2 cups water
Lavender essential oil (optional)

To a clean jar, add vinegar and lavender, and let the mixture sit for a few days, at which point you will notice the mixture turn a bright-pink color. Strain out the flower buds, and discard or compost.

To a clean 12-ounce spray bottle, add ½ cup lavender vinegar, and fill the bottle with water (about 1 cup). Shake gently to mix. If you desire a stronger scent, add a few drops of lavender essential oil.

To use: Spray cleaner on your coop surfaces and wipe them clean. Use this cleaner weekly to maintain a healthy chicken environment.

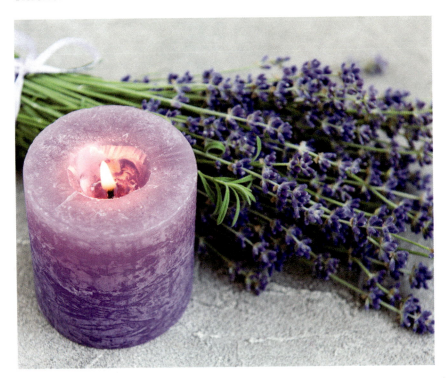

Lavender-Scented Candles

If you are new to candle making, this simple craft project requires a few simple ingredients and common kitchen equipment. Seasoned candle-makers can add lavender buds and oil to a favorite candle-making recipe.

To avoid ruining good pots and pans, dedicate a few old pots to the process. Yard sales and thrift stores are great places to find used kitchen equipment. For candle molds, I use everything

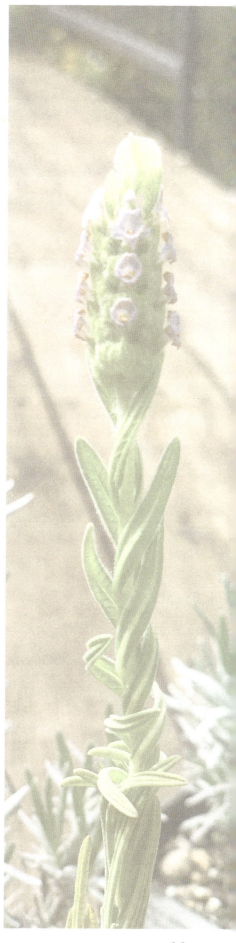

from old teacups, to terra cotta flower pots, tin cans, and old wax-lined food cartons. In lieu of using cotton string, purchase wicks from a craft store; your candles will burn much better. The number of candles yielded will depend on your mold size.

Yield: 16 ounces of wax

> **2 pounds beeswax, soy, or paraffin wax**
> **1 cup dried lavender buds or 2 cups fresh flowers**
> **5 to 6 drops lavender essential oil (optional)**
> **Coconut oil**
> **Candle mold**
> **Candle wick**

Break or chop up the beeswax into smaller pieces. Place the wax in a double boiler, or a pot set inside a pan of water, on the stovetop. Never melt your wax directly on the burner; always insulate it with a water bath. Keep the heat low so the wax melts slowly. Once it is completely melted, add the lavender, and stir well.

Prepare the molds by greasing them with a bit of coconut oil. Hang your wick from a skewer placed horizontally across the top of the mold. Alternately, if your wick comes with an adhesive, stick it to the bottom of the container. Stir wax until it starts to thicken, but is still pourable. Slowly pour wax into molds. Save a small amount to fill in around the wick when the wax dips in the center while cooling. Allow the wax to harden for several hours or overnight. Remove candle from mold .

Lavender Wands

The French tradition of making lavender wands, or bouteilles, will keep your drawers and closets smelling sweet. They also make lovely gifts. It is important to use freshly picked, long-stemmed lavender; it's more pliable and easier to work with. Long-stemmed varieties such as 'Grosso' or 'Provence' work well.

> **Odd number of lavender stems (I like to use 13)**
> **2 yards of ⅜-inch-wide ribbon**
> **Safety pin (optional)**

Gather lavender stalks and tie them together tightly with ribbon just under the flower heads. Turn your bundle so the flower heads are facing toward you. Gently

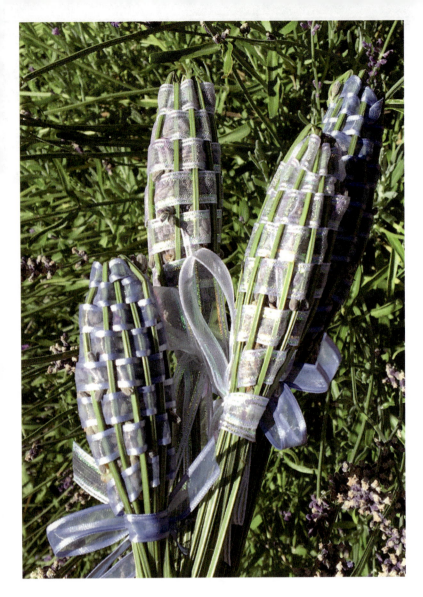

bend one stem at a time over the bundle of flower heads, and repeat until all of the stems are covering the flowers. Attach a safety pin to the end of a ribbon to give you something to hold onto, and weave ribbon perpendicular to the stems, over and under. This creates a sort of basket around the blooms to contain them after they dry. Continue weaving until the entire bundle is covered, and finally, tie the end of the ribbon around stems. Take a bit more ribbon and tie a bow at the base. Cut the stalks evenly to your desired wand length, and tie another bow around the stalks if necessary. For a simpler version, bend the stalks over the flower heads and tie a ribbon around the bent stalks without weaving.

To use: Place lavender wands next to your bed or in a drawer or closet. To refresh the scent, gently squeeze the woven end.

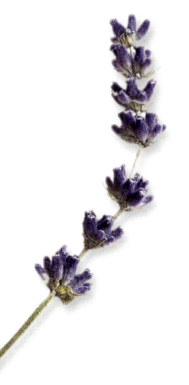

Lavender Sachets

These small, multi-purpose, scented pillows lend themselves to reusing and preserving some of your favorite fabrics. Preserve beloved clothing fabrics by making them into sachets that can be popped in a drawer or suitcase, or placed under a pillow at night. Wondering what to do with the beautiful monogrammed handkerchiefs my grandmother and great-grandmother handed down to me, I realized I could make them into lavender sachets. Feel free to create your own herbal blends, and sew your sachets into any shape you choose. My friend Lori makes her's into heart shapes that she tosses in the dryer to make her clothes smell amazing. If you are not into sewing, you can also use a good fabric glue, or even purchase ready-made

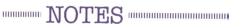
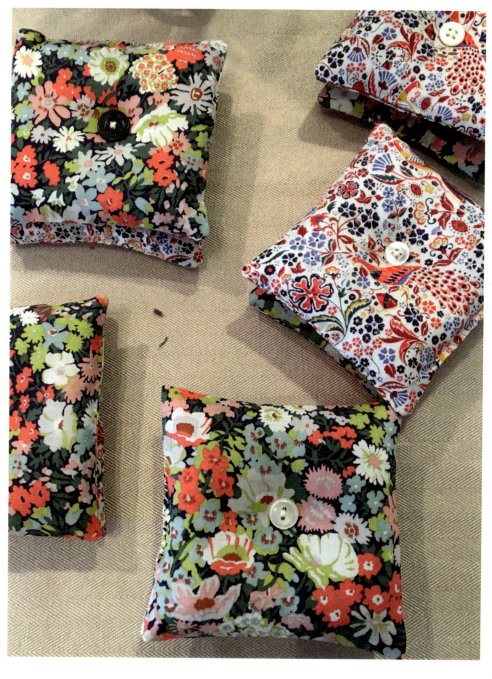

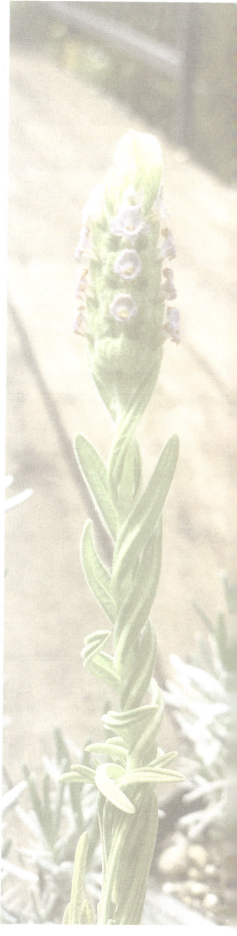

muslin drawstring bags available in tea shops to make sachets. **Yield: 1 square sachet**

¼ to ½ cup dried lavender buds
Clean cotton fabric
Cotton thread

Cut 2 squares of fabric any size you like. (Use the pattern on Page 103 or create your own.)

For a 4-inch square sachet, cut two squares 4½ inches with a seam allowance of a quarter inch on each side. With right sides together, stitch your fabric together, leaving a 1- to 2-inch opening. Turn inside-out and, over a large bowl or basket, fill sachets with dried lavender buds. Stitch the opening closed, and decorate the exterior with buttons or patches.

Sachet Ideas

Once you have mastered the basic sachet, get creative. Lavender sachets are useful around the house; they not only make things smell fresh while helping you relax, they also help keep away insects that may want to nibble on natural fabrics such as wool, cotton, or silk. They also absorb odors in shoes and suitcases with a little activated charcoal or cedar wood shavings added to the mix. Here is a brief list of uses:

Shoe inserts: Make foot-shaped sachets and fill with lavender, baking soda, and charcoal to absorb odors, and place them inside your shoes and garden boots.

Teddy bear bows: It's hard to clean whole dolls and teddy bears filled with lavender. Instead, to help small children relax, make a bow filled with herbs to place around a favorite toy. (See the pattern on Page 107.)

Closet hangers: Hang these with special clothing, such as wedding dresses and tuxedos. Trace a wood or metal hanger to create a large sachet that fits the body of the hanger. Fill with lavender and sew or glue in place. Or, simply tie a small sachet onto your hanger.

Suitcases: Place sachets inside totes, purses, and suitcases to keep them smelling fresh. Add optional baking soda, charcoal, or cedar wood shavings to the mix.

Dryer balls: Create simple sachets for tossing into your dryer with your clothes to keep things smelling fresh.

Pet beds: Make a small sachet to place on the bottom or inside of a pet bed to deter fleas and ticks. Do not use too much lavender, because some pets are sensitive to strong smells. If you find your pet avoiding its bed, you may want to remove or reduce the amount of lavender.

Dream pillows: Place small pillows filled with lavender, chamomile, and hops beside your bed or under your pillow for a restful night's sleep and sweet dreams. (See the Dream Pillows pattern on Page 104.)

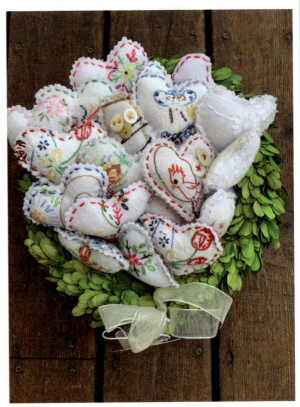

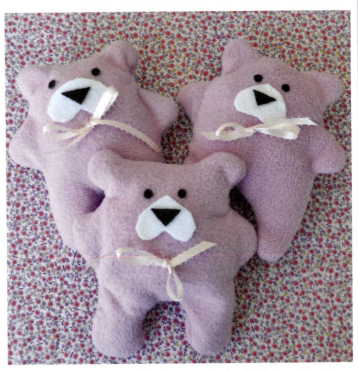

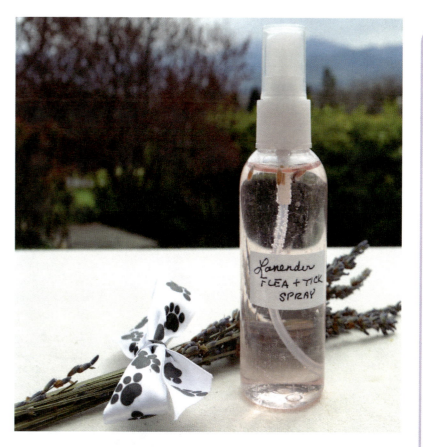

Lavender Flea and Tick Spray

Mix up this lavender spray for your special pet. It not only relaxes them and makes them smell good, it also safely and effectively repels pests. If you have questions, consult your vet before using. Some recipes use essential oils, and these work too, as long as you dilute your oils, and never use them directly on your pet or in their food. **Yield: 8 ounces**

    2 tablespoons witch hazel
    2 tablespoons apple cider vinegar or Lavender Vinegar (Page 43)
    1 cup strong Lavender Tea (1 tablespoon dried lavender to 1 cup water) (Page 75)

Mix together all ingredients, and pour into a clean spray bottle. Give the bottle a shake to mix well.

To use: Carefully spray the legs and bodies of pets, being careful not to spray near their heads, eyes, noses, or mouths.

To apply the spray to your pet's neck, soak a cotton bandana or washcloth in the solution, and rub all over the neck area. You can leave the bandana around your pet's neck until it is dry. Remove if they run outdoors. Use this spray to disinfect their beds and furniture to repel fleas.

Lavender and Pets

Lavender is a popular ingredient in natural flea and tick products sold in pet stores. Here are a few other ways you can use lavender as a natural remedy in your home:

• Grow lavender in your yard. If your dogs and cats like to spend time outdoors, they can pick up fleas and bring them into your house. Growing lavender plants in areas that they frequent brings beauty to your yard while warding off fleas and ticks.

• Give your pet a Lavender Salt (Page 66) bath. Bath soaks are not just for us humans. Keep the water temperature cool, using ½ cup salt in a bathtub half-full of water. The salt water will dehydrate any fleas and kill them off. Rinse your dog well after a salt bath as the salt also dehydrates your pet's skin.

• Brush your pet's fur with a dry brush sprinkled with some diluted lavender essential oil. Never use undiluted essential oils on your pets; instead, create a scented oil by mixing a few drops essential oil into ¼ cup olive or grapeseed oil. Sprinkle a dry pet brush with the oil mixture, and use it to groom your dog or cat. The oil will help comb out any pests and leave your pet with a shiny coat.

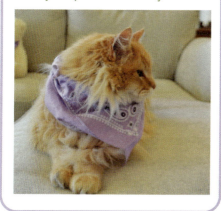

Lavender Potpourri Dishes

Potpourri dishes are gaining popularity. Instead of the old wood shavings and dusty dried flowers, potpourri is now filled with scented, colorful herbs and flowers arranged in an artful way in pretty dishes on bedside tables, bathroom counters, or coffee tables for handling and sparking conversation.

To keep potpourri safe from spills, place it in a canning jar with a screened lid, and gently shake the jar to release the scent. **Yield: 16 ounces**

1 to 2 cups dried lavender buds and leaves

½ teaspoon orris root powder
Dried petals of 3 to 4 roses, calendulas, geraniums, or citrus peels (or a combination of your favorites)
Lavender essential oil (optional)

Place the lavender buds and orris root powder in a bowl, and mix well. The orris root powder acts as a fixative so your potpourri lasts longer. For a stronger scent, add a few drops of lavender essential oil. Place the lavender in a small bowl or decorative dish. Then arrange your other dried plant materials in a design that is pleasing to you. I find this to be a relaxing, almost meditative craft.

History of Potpourri

Since ancient times, potpourri has been scattered on floors, or placed around rooms in pots with perforated lids. It has traditionally been made with freshly cut spring herbs and flowers, layered with salt, and laid out to dry during the summer months. In the fall, spices and fixatives such as orris root would be added until the scent was pleasing. The mixtures were then placed around the home in bowls or in ceramic containers to perfume the air. Dried potpourri mixes can last from two months to 20 years, depending on storage and the plant material used. Some home décor shops sell potpourri mixes made of wood shavings, plant materials, and synthetic scents. These are not traditional potpourris in my opinion; nothing beats using real natural plant material. Of course, lavender remains a popular potpourri plant among the 300 different plant species used throughout history.

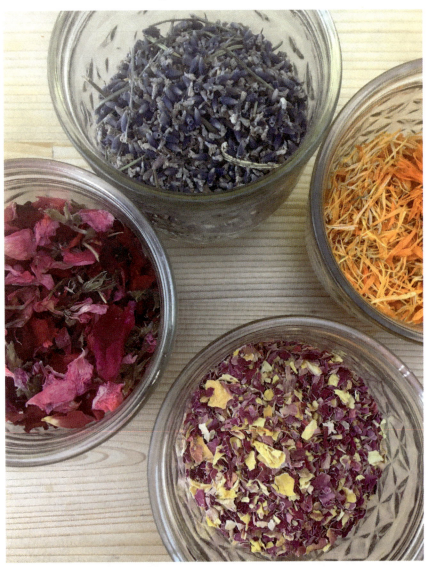

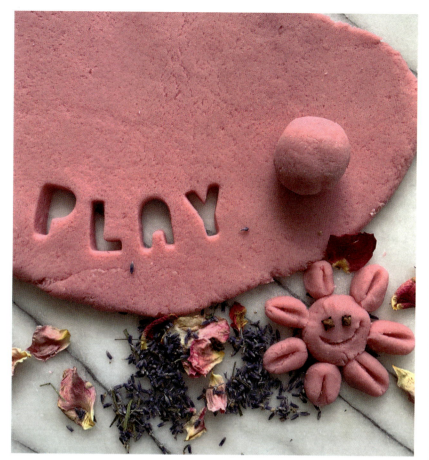

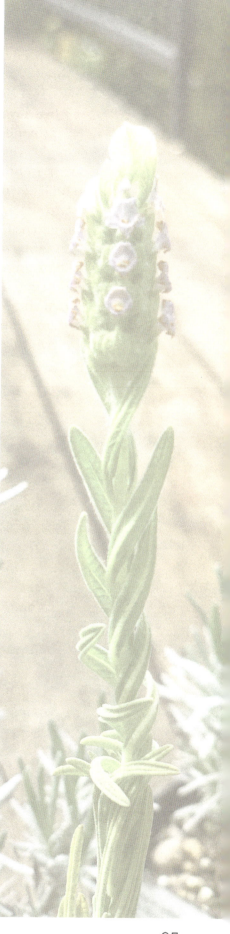

Lavender-Scented Play Dough

I started using this recipe when my daughters were in preschool for a creative and calming activity at home. That was almost 30 years ago, and I find myself making it still today for people of all ages. It is non-toxic, so don't worry if it drops on the ground and the dog eats it. Though we made this dough one year for a workshop as a kids craft, I noticed the adults having just as much fun with it. Red hibiscus tea gives the dough a hot-pink hue, and blue butterfly pea tea gives it a purple shade. Have fun experimenting with other natural colors and scents. **Yield: 8 ounces**

    1 cup flour
    ½ cup salt
    1 cup hot water or strong herbal tea
    1 tablespoon sunflower or vegetable oil
    2 teaspoons cream of tartar
    2 to 3 drops lavender essential oil (optional)
    2 tablespoons dried lavender leaves and flowers (optional)

Mix together the flour, salt, tea, oil, and cream of tartar in a saucepan. Heat for 1 to 2 minutes over low heat. Remove the pan from the heat, and stir in the essential oil and dried lavender.

Place the dough on a lightly floured board, and knead until smooth. Store in an airtight container.

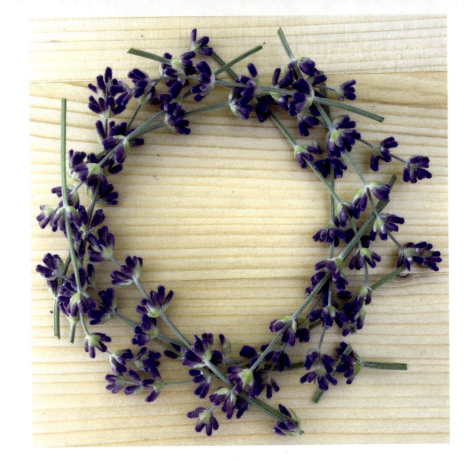

Uses for Lavender Stems

Use your sturdy lavender stems as bamboo skewers and toothpicks. Cut them to the desired length, let dry, and store them in jars. Be sure to soak them first before using as grill skewers, or before adding to your smoker to flavor meats. Lavender stems can also be woven into small baskets with the same method as pine-needle baskets. Gather small bunches of stems and secure with garden twine or raffia in a circular pattern.

The stems also add a bit of texture to wreaths and foraged floral arrangements. If you have a large amount of stems, place them in chicken coops, boxes, or stalls as bedding. The subtle scent of the stems keeps pests away and helps calm your livestock.

Lavender Wreaths and Crowns

Decorate your home year-round with a lavender wreath, or wear it as a crown! Use freshly harvested lavender with new or "tight" buds to keep your wreath intact. Use fresh, pliable lavender so the wreath dries in place. Hang or store your freshly made wreath in a place with good airflow and out of direct sunlight to keep the colors bright. If you need more lavender than you have in your garden, visit a local farm when the flowers are at full bloom. Many farms offer U-pick prices, and some even have wreath-making classes as an activity during the summer months. **Yield: 1 wreath**

1 paddle of floral wire
Wire wreath form or grapevine form
Freshly harvested lavender with tight buds
Ribbon for decoration (optional)
Other freshly harvest herbs (optional)
Small hand pruners or sharp scissors

Attach your floral wire to the wreath form. Gather small bunches of about 20 to 30 lavender stems in your hand, and trim the stems. Place your first bunch on the wreath form, and secure with floral wire. Wrap the bunch a few times to secure it, since the bunches will shrink a bit when dried.

Take a second bunch, and layer it on top of the first one, covering the stems with the flower heads. Secure the second bunch with wire, and repeat with more flower

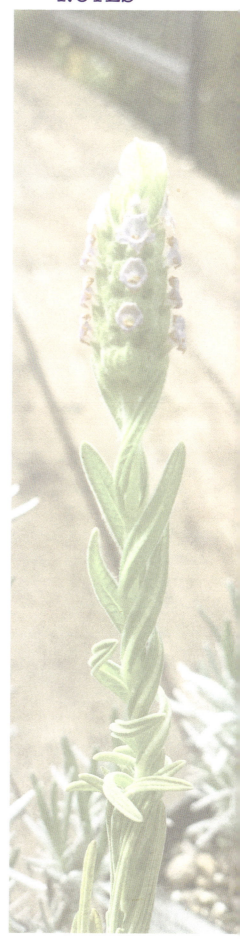

bunches until you have worked your way around the form. Secure your wire and tuck all the stems under the flower heads. If you are pleased with your wreath, decorate it with a fabric or raffia bow, and tuck in other herbs and flowers, such as rosemary or roses.

If you want a fuller wreath, repeat the steps, and go around your form one more time with more bunches of lavender.

Add a bit of string or wire on the back of your wreath for hanging.

To use: Hang your wreath in a dry spot with good airflow, out of direct sunlight.

Lavender Fire Starters

After de-budding your lavender (see Page 32), you will be left with a large quantity of stems. These have a more subtle scent than the flower heads and contain less oil, yet they still smell like lavender. You can make fire starters for your home, or to start a campfire with the scented kindling. Bind them with raffia or cotton string that can be burned.

> **50 dried lavender stems**
> **Raffia or garden twine**
> **Pruning shears or scissors**

Gather up your lavender stems, and tie them securely on each end and in the middle with a bit of twine or raffia. With sharp scissors or pruning shears, trim the ends over a bucket or basket for a more uniform bunch.

To use: Place in your fireplace as you would kindling and light to start a fire.

Aromatherapy Charms and Bracelets

Scented jewelry has been popular since ancient times. Queen Nefertiti of Egypt was well-known for carrying a scented sachet tied at her waist during the 18th dynasty. My grandmother had a similar pendant that she wore around her neck, filled with scented tablets. Today's aromatherapy jewelry not only makes you smell nice; it also helps create a mood for the wearer. They are super simple to create, all you need are some basic craft supplies: lava stone or wooden beads and air-dry clay.

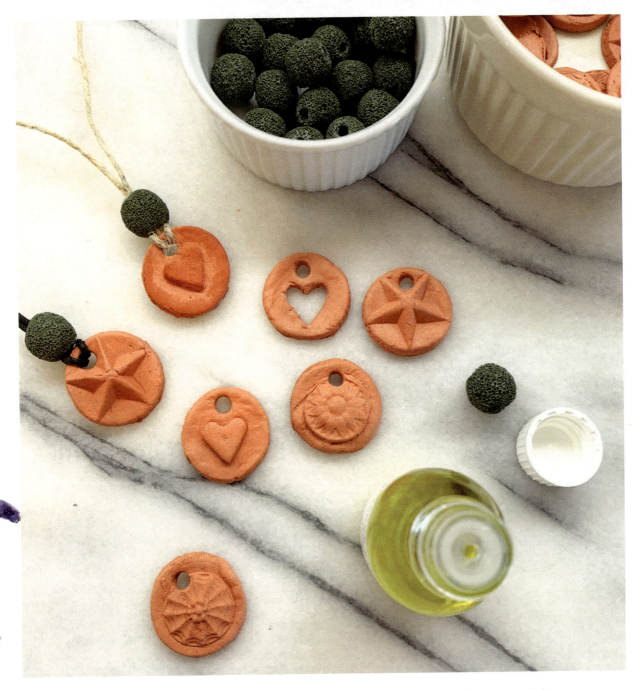

All of these materials are found at most craft stores. The porous materials soak up the scented essential oil and slowly release the scent as your body warms the jewelry. They are also a nice gift to make and fun to create.

Lava stone beads or natural wood beads
Air-hardening natural clay
String

Clay-Working Tools:
Small roller
Cookie cutters
Bottle caps
Stamps

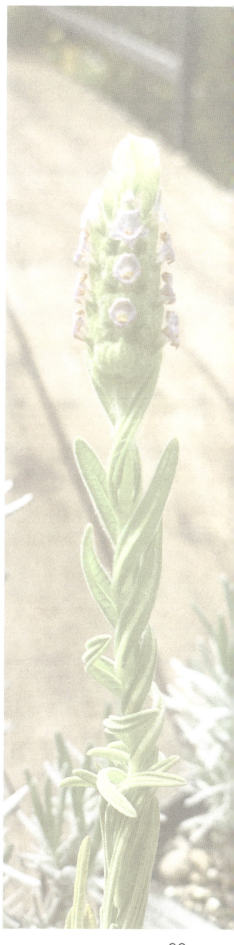

To make the clay charms, roll out clay, cut it into the shape you like, make a small hole for hanging the charm, and let it dry overnight. I use a bottle cap to cut out small circles, and I decorate them with a small stamp or make an impression with a sturdy leaf or flower head.

To create pendants and bracelets, string a lava bead, clay charm, and any other charms onto a string or elastic band. To plan your design, lay them out on a plate before stringing.

To use: Apply a drop or two of scented oil or oil blend to the porous beads and charms. Depending on how often you wear your jewelry, reapply oil as needed. I store mine in a small jar to keep the scent from fading.

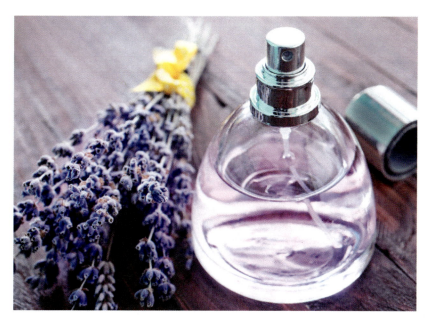

Lavender Linen Spray

Many hotels now provide a small vial of lavender water next to the bed, allowing guests to spray it on their pillows or sheets to help them wind down naturally for a good night's sleep. Use this scented water in your iron to press fine linens, and for spraying generously onto your bed pillow each evening. **Yield: 4 ounces**

½ **cup purified water**
1 **teaspoon vodka or witch hazel**
5 **to 6 drops lavender essential oil**

Mix all ingredients together, and pour into a clean spray bottle or glass container with a tight-fitting lid.

Recipes, Notes, and Ingredient Sources

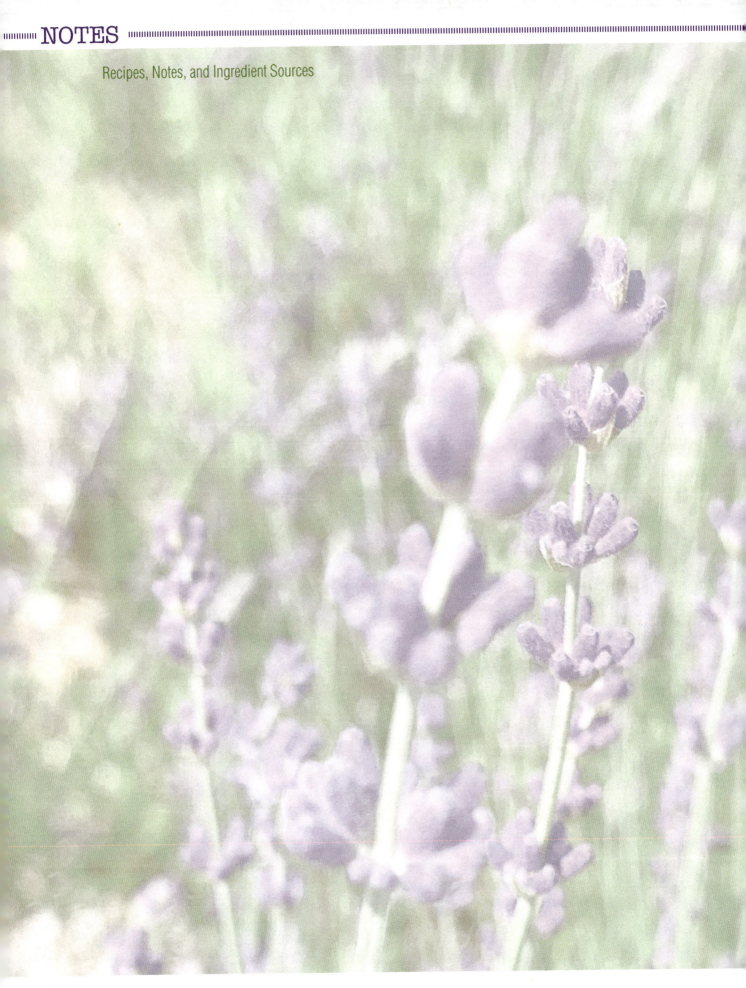

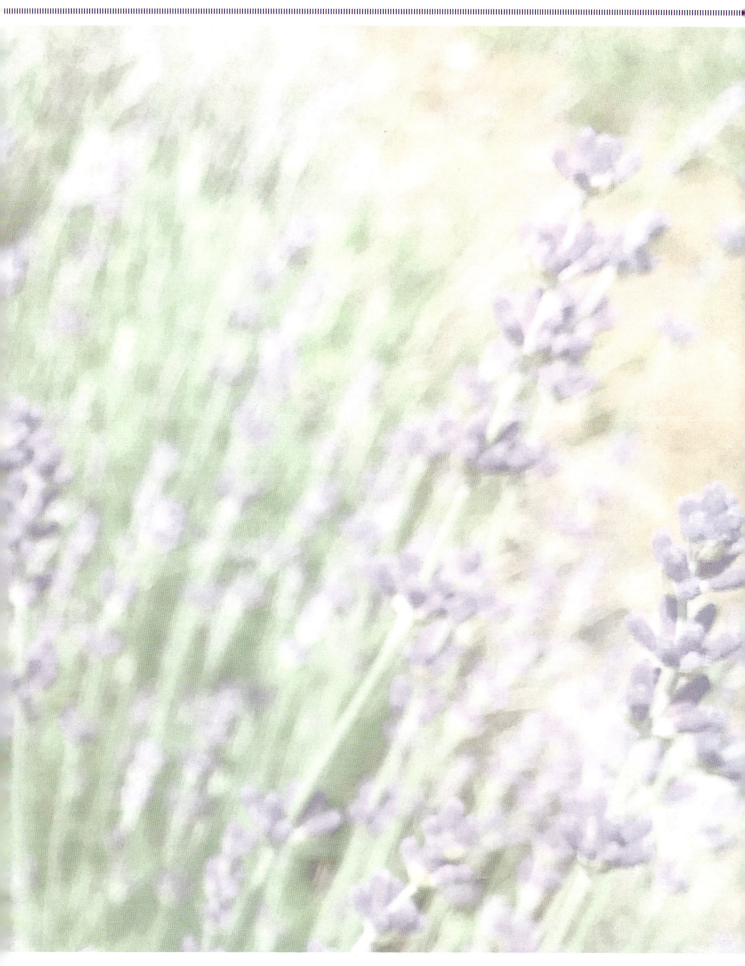

Creating your own lavender products is a wonderful way to expand your personal health-care and body-care tools. Another plus with making these products is the opportunity for great gift-giving ideas.

On the following pages, you will find templates and instructions to make a Basic Sachet Pattern (below) for the Lavender Sachets on Page 90; the invitation for the tea party mentioned on Page 76 (using the recipes and blends found on Pages 74 and 75); the Lavender Dream Pillows described on Page 59; the Eye Rest Pillow that begins on Page 58; and the Lavender Bear and the Teddy Bear Bow (Sachets) Patterns spotlighted on Page 92.

Whatever recipe or pattern you select for your next project, you will know the product meets your exacting standards and that it will fill your life with the benefits and scent of lavender!

BASIC SACHET PATTERN

¼-inch seam

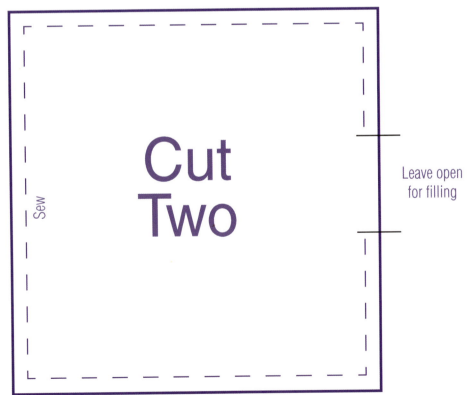

Sew

Cut
Two

Leave open
for filling

4-inch square

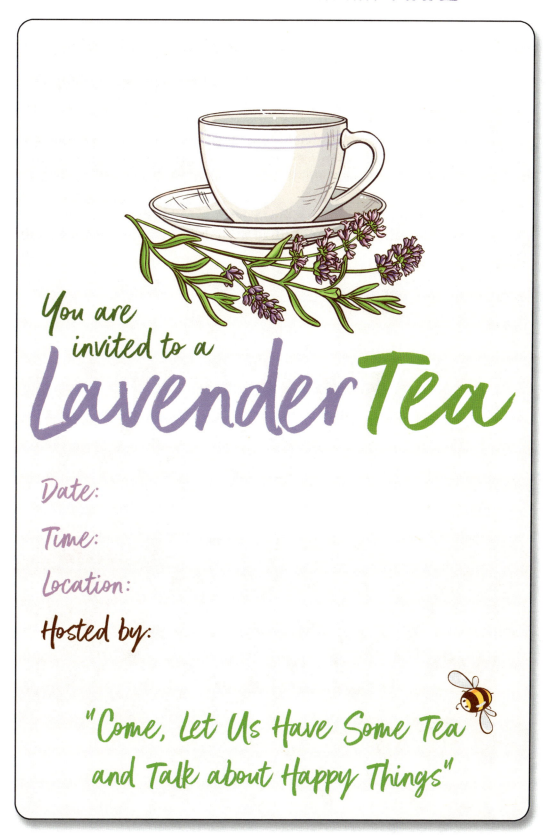

You are
invited to a

Lavender Tea

Date:

Time:

Location:

Hosted by:

"Come, Let Us Have Some Tea
and Talk about Happy Things"

DREAM PILLOW PATTERN
(Drawstring Bag)

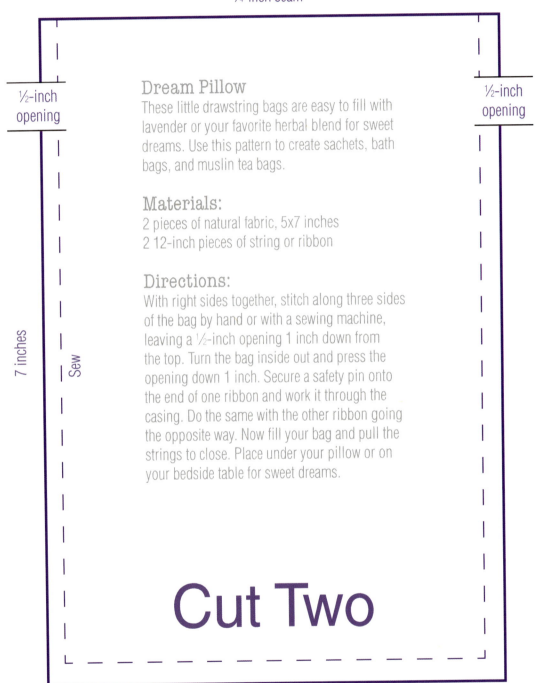

¼-inch seam

½-inch opening

½-inch opening

7 inches

Sew

Dream Pillow
These little drawstring bags are easy to fill with lavender or your favorite herbal blend for sweet dreams. Use this pattern to create sachets, bath bags, and muslin tea bags.

Materials:
2 pieces of natural fabric, 5x7 inches
2 12-inch pieces of string or ribbon

Directions:
With right sides together, stitch along three sides of the bag by hand or with a sewing machine, leaving a ½-inch opening 1 inch down from the top. Turn the bag inside out and press the opening down 1 inch. Secure a safety pin onto the end of one ribbon and work it through the casing. Do the same with the other ribbon going the opposite way. Now fill your bag and pull the strings to close. Place under your pillow or on your bedside table for sweet dreams.

Cut Two

5 inches

EYE REST PILLOW PATTERN

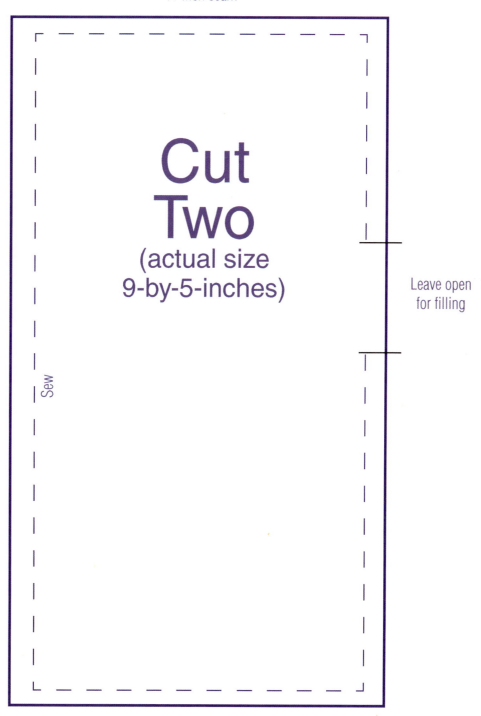

¼-inch seam

Cut
Two
(actual size
9-by-5-inches)

Leave open
for filling

Sew

Enlarge at 125% on a photocopier
to create the full-size pillow pattern.

LAVENDER BEAR PATTERN

FOLD

Cut Two

Leave open
for filling

Sew
2 pieces together

Nose A
Cut 1

Stuff with cotton and lavender

Eyes

Nose B
Cut 1

TEDDY BEAR BOW (SACHET) PATTERN

Teddy Bear Bows

Materials:
1 to 2 tablespoons dried lavender
1 10-inch ribbon
1 12-inch elastic

Directions:
1. Cut out two bow pieces using the pattern.
2. With the right sides pinned together, stitch around all edges leaving a 1-inch gap on one side for filling. Turn right side out.
3. Fill the bow with the lavender, or use cotton batting. Close the opening by hand stitching.
4. Tie the ends of the elastic to form a loop.
5. Use the ribbon to form the bow shape and to fasten the bow to the elastic.
6. Place the elastic and bow around the neck of your favorite stuffed animal. (See photo on Page 84.)

Note: Teddy bear bows can also be used on hat bands, baskets, and packages; anywhere you may want a bit of calming lavender scent.

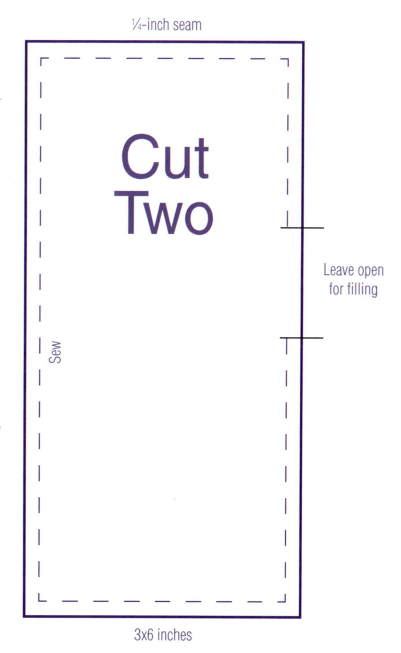

¼-inch seam

Cut Two

Sew

Leave open for filling

3x6 inches

Index

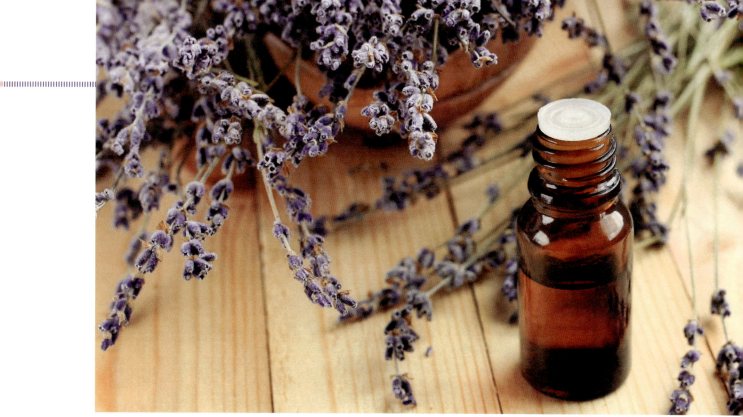

Index

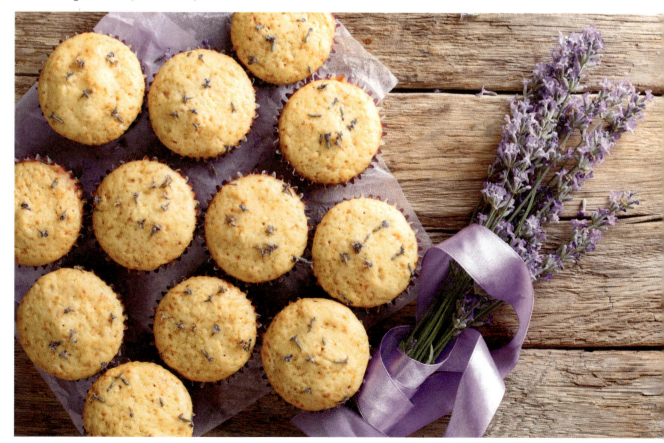

Photo Credits

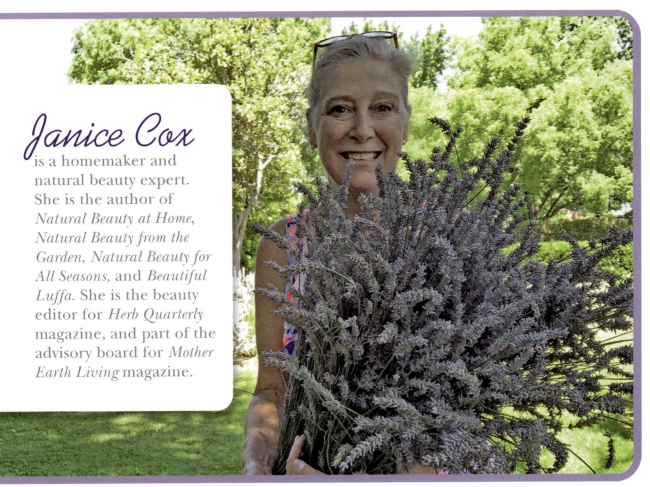

Janice Cox

is a homemaker and natural beauty expert. She is the author of *Natural Beauty at Home, Natural Beauty from the Garden, Natural Beauty for All Seasons,* and *Beautiful Luffa.* She is the beauty editor for *Herb Quarterly* magazine, and part of the advisory board for *Mother Earth Living* magazine.